Emotion Rituals

Emotion Rituals

A resource for therapists and clients

David W. McMillan

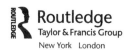

Routledge
Taylor & Francis Group
New York London

Published in 2006 by
Routledge
Taylor & Francis Group
711 Third Avenue
New York, NY 10017

Published in Great Britain by
Routledge
Taylor & Francis Group
27 Church Road
Hove, East Sussex BN3 2FA

© 2006 by Taylor & Francis Group, LLC
Routledge is an imprint of Taylor & Francis Group

First issued in paperback 2013

International Standard Book Number-13: 978-0-415-86120-5 (pbk)
International Standard Book Number-13: 978-0-415-95209-5 (hbk)
Library of Congress Card Number 2005017179

Library of Congress Cataloging-in-Publication Data

McMillan, David W.
    Emotion rituals : a resource for therapists and clients / David W. McMillan.
        p. cm.
    Includes bibliographical references and index.
    ISBN 0-415-95209-3
    1. Cognitive therapy. 2. Emotions--Therapeutic use. 3. Ritual--Therapeutic use. 4. Psychotherapy.
I. Title.

RC489.C63M345 2005
616.89'142--dc22
                                                          2005017179

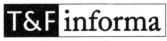

Taylor & Francis Group
is the Academic Division of T&F Informa plc.

Visit the Taylor & Francis Web site at
http://www.taylorandfrancis.com

and the Routledge Web site at
http://www.routledge-ny.com

To my wife, Marietta,
who has taught me more
about emotions than
any person on earth.

Contents

Preface

Cognitive behavioral psychotherapy currently is the most popular theory in psychotherapy education and practice. The basic assumption of the theory is that illogical thoughts create pathological behavior and dysfunction. On one hand, this approach is beneficial because it provides concrete practical strategies for treating psychological problems. On the other hand, the most often repeated criticism of this treatment approach is that it ignores emotions (Atkinson, 1999; Greenberg, 2001).

As cognitive behavioral theory suggests, thoughts can change feelings. But feelings also can change feelings, and imagination can create feelings. Take music as an example. Say each emotion is like a musical note. Played consecutively, these notes can produce a pleasing melody. But when a musical composition monotonously repeats one note, again and again, the result can drive us crazy.

In real life, seldom do we feel a single emotion for a long period of time. Moving rhythmically forward, one emotion is followed by another and then another, creating a flow of many emotions. When we are able to do this, we say we are in a healthy state. But when we are stuck in one feeling—or when there is but one repetitive note and no rhythm—pathology takes over.

This is not a new thought. Theorists from Freud to Rogers have said the same thing. This book introduces two new ideas. The first is that it is not enough to simply unblock emotions. There are times when emotions need to be contained. The goal of psychotherapy should be to help clients master their emotions. *Emotion Rituals* gives the therapist tools to help clients achieve emotional awareness and control.

The second new idea presented in this book is that each discrete emotion has its own dynamic. Psychotherapists can make use of the dynamics of the individual discrete emotion to help restore a healthy flow of emotions.

The new idea we present is that by using the resources in each discrete emotion as a therapeutic resource, we can create therapeutic rituals for clients. Psychotherapists have done a credible job of helping frightened and sad clients access their innate strong emotions of desire and anger to assert their way out of anxiety and depression. But psychotherapists have done a poor job of helping angry or manic individuals discover a healthy emotional balance; or helping happy, arrogant, self-absorbed individuals become accountable and respectful; or helping shame-filled, dramatic, self-destructive individuals find a more positive view of themselves.

This book offers therapeutic rituals, using imagination and discrete emotions to restore a healthy emotional flow. These rituals can help us get out of the traps that each emotion can create, offering remedies for each emotional dysfunction.

The therapeutic techniques introduced in *Emotion Rituals* are like those of cognitive behavioral therapy in that they involve self-talk. It is distinct from cognitive behavioral therapy in that the self-talk used here is a ritual, not a lecture. Its focus is emotions, not ideas or self-judgments. While cognitive behavioral therapy teaches a person to process critical life events rationally, the emotion exercises proposed in *Emotion Rituals* are aimed at changing brain chemicals, shifting neurological paths, and rebalancing a person's emotional climate. The rituals suggested here can be used once or twice a day or more often, like meditation or prayer. Or, they can be used as needed. They can be used to help clients adapt to difficult moments, but that is not their raison d'être. Rituals slowly build new emotional paths toward inner harmony and strength. They can move us out of emotional knots, cycles, and traps and into a healthy emotional flow.

In conceiving *Emotion Rituals,* I intended it to be a serious text for students, scholars, and practitioners of psychotherapy. *Emotion Rituals* might serve as a second text in an introductory psychotherapy class (supplementing a primary text that would teach students how to listen). Included in this book is a section dedicated to the neuro-physiological basis of emotion. This section grounds the clinical ideas in the book in brain research and physiology. Some readers might wish to skip this section and proceed to the more practice-oriented section of the book.

My goal is to share with the reader the sense of excitement and discovery I experienced as I began to explore how emotions flow together. Such a simple idea and yet so useful to psychotherapy: each emotion can resolve other emotions!

The psychotherapist who works with emotions in this way is not simply a cognitive behavioral therapist or a client-centered therapist. Using emotions as psychotherapeutic tools is much like prescribing medication and watching clients improve. Why? Because emotions are tied to our brains and our biochemicals. Brain chemicals communicate with each other and change one another. When our emotions change, our brain chemistry changes, too. If they know what they are doing, therapists can help clients change their brain chemistry just as Prozac can.

The point of *Emotion Rituals* is that we can change our neurochemistry ourselves without taking drugs. We can change our brain chemistry by changing the way we process our emotions. The therapist can help clients choose the neurohormone and neurotransmitter exchanges that clients prefer by leading them through an emotional process that turns on different neurocircuits and creates new brain chemical reactions.

How This Book Is Organized

The opening chapters of this book familiarize readers with the lineage of the book's theory, its historical and philosophical roots. In these chapters, readers also will become familiar with the workings of the brain and neurohormones, neurological language, and the neuroanatomy of each emotion. I introduce this by using conversations that have occurred during consultation group meetings. I framed the book's theoretical roots and the neurology of the theory in this conversational style for several reasons. One is that such collegial settings offer great opportunities for support and learning. Many readers of this book will be familiar with exchanges of this type. Second, these ideas and the language in which they are expressed can be intimidating. Conversational language makes them less so. Three, when I write as if I'm talking my ideas are clearer to me as well.

After this initiation into emotion theory and emotion neurology, the book begins to explore how the therapist can guide clients out of unhealthy emotional patterns into healthy emotional flows. At this point, therapists will be on familiar ground and can begin to generate their own ideas and theories.

To make this theory accessible, I write as if emotions operate linearly. They don't. The brain rarely feels just one thing. Several emotions co-exist concurrently in our brains, just as great music has texts and subtexts playing at the same time.

One emotion may be dominant, but it is certainly not alone. Remembering that many emotions can occur together is an important caveat in reading this book. Perhaps a later theorist will describe how these multi-layered emotions work together—experientially and chemically—and psychotherapists can help clients write complex emotional symphonies, instead of merely discovering simple emotional melodies, as I have done here. This is the promise of this theory and this book: its purpose is to introduce the emotion flow and explain how therapists can use discrete emotions to help people feel better.

The Anatomy of a Psychological Theory

To build a psychological theory, one must explain its effect on psychology's holy trinity: thinking, feeling, and behaving. Often, just covering the bases of thinking and behaving is enough. In this book, however, I want to emphasize the importance of feelings in any theory that explains the human psyche. And I hope to raise the bar by transforming this holy trinity into a holy quartet: feeling, thinking, behaving, and neurologically interacting.

Now that we know so much about the brain and how it functions, we mental health professionals must include neurological circuitry and brain chemistry in our theories of how humans function. We know that thoughts, feelings, and behavior have neurological markers. Feelings include chemical exchanges of neuromodulating chemicals. I propose that we can change how we feel through chemistry.

Managed care has forced us to include quicker, less intensive techniques in our therapeutic repertoire. While obviously following this path has contributed to increasing the repertoire of skills of the therapist, these techniques are only useful to perhaps one-half or less of clients typical of a psychotherapy practice. And these techniques are not useful at all to the therapist who does not know how to build a therapeutic alliance with the client. Empathy and active listening skills remain essential therapeutic tools.

This book is not, however, primarily about building the therapeutic alliance. Rather, it provides a theory base for a new set of psychotherapy tools that have an extensive theoretical and neurological foundation. The therapeutic alliance is the context for these tools.

This is the first of several books I hope to write using the same emotion theory base. The theory applies Tomkins' (1963) emotions theory to practical clinical work. In my application of this theory, I contend that we are always feeling something. Most of the time, we are in emotional steady states such as mild interest or contentment. Daily, sometimes momentarily, our feelings shift from one to the other depending on the circumstances we confront.

The Significance of Neurology to Behavioral Treatment

I contend that we have nine basic emotions: anger, fear, sadness, shame, desire, joy, surprise, fatigue, and disgust. According to Tomkins (1963), each of our emotions serves an adaptive purpose. We need to use all of them from time to time and at varying levels of intensity.

Psychopathology occurs when we get stuck in one emotion or in an emotional knot or cycle. When we are emotionally trapped in this way, we need to discover healthy paths to help us out of the psychopathology of emotional paralysis.

After finishing this book, readers should be able to understand and teach others how emotions work. I hope readers will be able to give concrete, specific ideas to clients that will help clients function better in their daily lives. Many of these ideas are new. Some are not. But the theory that unites them is intended to be common-sensical and constructive.

Parenthetically, this theory explains the neurology of cognitive behavioral treatment. Primarily, it unites art, imagination, emotions, and neurobiology into a theory that gives practical concrete rituals, which clients can follow. With practice, clients will feel the change. Self-esteem and strength will come from building their own emotional skills. *Emotion Rituals* provides the basis for a new set of clinical tools that use basic discrete emotions.

Writing Voices

This book speaks to the reader in several voices: a clinical, case study voice, which is authentically mine and is akin to a southern story-telling voice; a conversational theoretical voice, which is my voice and the voice of my colleagues; a voice of a scholastic reporter describing the neurobiology of the brain and adopting the tone of a heavy, neuropsychology-journal article.

The case-study voice is meant to help the reader apply the theory practically. The conversational theory voice aims to make the complex clearer and more understandable. The reporter voice attempts to help the reader identify the parts of the brain along with the brain's neurohormones that therapists might hope to change when using these ideas in therapy.

In chapters 1 and 2, I use the consulting group context to introduce the logical underpinnings of the theory. Chapter 3 moves between the scholastic-reporter voice and the story-telling voice, introducing the reader to the, perhaps, foreign world of neuroanatomy. I hope this sometimes dense chapter will help familiarize the therapist with what is happening in clients' brains as we attempt to help them change. The story-telling voice and the theory-building voice alternate in the remaining chapters.

Most of the ideas I present are introduced, explained, and summarized in clinical case studies. Of course, these are not true stories. Only those stories in which I am the main character have any semblance of reality. But they are the compilation of thousands of voices and circumstances that have been part of my clinical practice.

The Energy Patterns of Emotions

Like musical notes, emotions can oppose as well as encourage one another. They can move tangentially and parallel to one another. They can work together to create a totally new emotional experience. Anger, fear, desire, disgust, and surprise all give the body energy, while sadness, shame, and fatigue/rest/sleep/trance withdraw energy.

Approach emotions create energy directed toward an object, e.g., desire and anger. Other emotions act to repel us, e.g., disgust, fear, and shame.

Some emotions have little movement, toward or away from; joy is one of these. It is what we express when we reach a goal. It is a destination emotion. Joy expresses victory, mastery, and relief of tension.

Surprise is neither an "approach" nor "avoid" emotion. It excites, but energy created by desire can use surprise to move toward, or energy created by fear can use surprise to move away from.

Still other emotions act in an either/or fashion. We can feel either fear or anger—but not both. We can feel sadness or anger—but not both; fatigue/rest/sleep/trance or fear—but not both; joy or sadness—but not both; joy or shame—but not both; fatigue/rest/sleep/trance or desire—but not both.

Some of these polar, either/or emotions provide healthy resolutions for one another. In this text, joy and shame is our most emphasized, resolving pair. Fear and anger resolve one another, but so what? Who wants to use fear as a resolve to anger, and anger is only perhaps a slight improvement on fear. While we want to use fatigue/rest/sleep/trance to resolve fear, only in a real crisis do we want fear to resolve fatigue/rest/sleep/trance.

Dissecting the Emotion Chapters

Chapter 5 is the first chapter to discuss a specific emotion, in this case anger. The following chapters, 6 through 13, each discuss one emotion and follow similar organization.

They begin with a definition of the emotion, followed by a clinical case study that puts the treatment of this emotion in context. This is followed by a review of the physiology and then the intelligence of that emotion. The next section describes the negative consequences of the emotion, followed by a discussion of the positive ones. Issues pertaining to that particular emotion are discussed in mid-chapter. The chapter continues with a discussion of how to resolve the emotion effectively. Next is a ritual to help clients find a healthy path out of the pathology that the emotion can create. The chapter ends with the conclusion of the story that introduced the chapter; it summarizes and resolves the emotional dilemma that the emotion creates.

And in Conclusion...

Chapter 14 describes the function and skills involved in empathy or compassion. Empathy uses every emotion and has a specific way of turning on the appropriate parts of the brain and releasing appropriate neurohormones.

Empathy is the most important tool in using emotions and connecting with the emotions of others. In the final chapter, I summarize the theory and suggest its potential uses in practice and its potential to change the way therapy currently is practiced.

The Role of the Reader

As I describe these emotions, I hope that my readers will take their turns at putting these relationships in some sort of a scheme with lines and arrows, colors, dots, or musical qualities. I hope that they will hear or imagine music that builds the healthy emotional paths I describe. By describing how emotions fit together, I show how each emotion is unique, yet possessing properties that link emotions to one another.

To understand these properties and how emotions collaborate with one another is to understand yourself and others. In this way, you can become the master of yourself. Instead of being stuck in an emotional fugue or driven out of control by internal, angry drumbeats, you can use your imagination to create new internal music and to create emotional harmony from discord. Absorbing and putting to use this information creates choices we never had before, as individuals or as therapists.

I had great fun writing *Emotion Rituals*. I hope my enthusiasm is evident, and I hope you enjoy reading it.

Acknowledgments

Thank yous seem so trite at this point. This project has been five years in the writing and many more years in the percolating of these ideas. No one person should be given credit for such an extensive project.

My wife, the Honorable Marietta Shipley, has listened, read, waited for me to finish another sentence, shared our vacations with my yellow pad and pen and my mind on my next chapter that I had to write. My deceased parents showed me emotional strength and courage, as they coped with the loss of their oldest son at age 19.

My mentor Bob Newbrough read the first draft of this book and encouraged me to believe that I could contribute to the discourse in psychotherapy. Jules Seeman read a draft and advised me to introduce each chapter with what I intended to say, to write it and then to conclude each chapter by recapping what I said.

Several colleagues read the manuscript and advised me. They are David Yarian, Larry Seeman, Linda Ramsey, Linda Stere, Peter Scanlan, Linda Wirth, Lynn Walker, and Jerome Burt. Hans Strupp also read a draft and encouraged me in this project. I am indebted to Jan Keeling, who helped me conceptualize this book by challenging me to find the good of shame. Michael Kaminski, M.D., helped me understand the biology of the brain; however, he is in no way responsible for any errors or oversimplifications that may be in the book. I am grateful for his time and attention.

Jason Link and Jenni Schaefer helped with research and editing. I am grateful to Susan Lewis for continually challenging my limited understanding of joy. And to my friend and colleague Stephen Prasinos for helping me understand that joy is an important part of compassion and community. I am the joyful recipient of the editing of Ann Granning Bennett and Lynn

Goeller. I am especially grateful to Gloria Schmittou for typing and retyping the manuscript.

I appreciate the ideas George Zimmar gave me that helped shape my ideas into this product. I am grateful to Larry Wrightsman, without whom I would not be a psychologist, and to Larry Weitz, who taught me how to listen. I am grateful to the introductory graduate psychotherapy class members at Tennessee State University and to Darrell Smith, their professor, for reading and reflecting on this work.

CHAPTER 1

A Simple Notion

It was the third Wednesday of March. The third Wednesday meant that my therapist consultation group was meeting. And March meant that I was scheduled to present.

I am always somewhat nervous when it is my turn. But this time I was more nervous than usual. I did not follow customary procedure by presenting an actual case for the consideration of my colleagues. Instead, I had sent my colleagues a draft of this book two weeks before the meeting, hoping it would provide a platform for discussion.

We have 10 members in our group; usually 5 show. As this was the public school spring break, our 10-member group became only 3, plus me, but this did not lessen my nervousness. Tom is a professor at Vanderbilt. He teaches family therapy as well as the history of psychology. Jane is a social worker, who sees the world through a New Age lens. She is always full of questions. Ralph is an analytic type who understands and appreciates object relations and psychodynamic theory. Ralph taught philosophy, before becoming a psychotherapist. All of them brought with them the blue plastic three-ring binder that contained the draft of this book.

Tom wasted no time. "So you've written your magnum opus, a treatise on why cognitive behavioral therapy is not enough."

"That's not his point," Ralph countered. "His point is that emotions have a dynamic, and each one has a different dynamic."

"Why don't we let David tell us the point of his book?" Jane suggested.

"Well, Tom and Ralph have it right," I said. "It is a simple notion that I had never heard of or thought about in my training. The notion is simply that feelings change feelings. As Tom said, cognitive behavioral theory leaves out emotion. I've never believed you could think your way sane. Yet, I appreciate how cognitive behavioral therapy has helped therapists be concrete, task

1

oriented, and behind what the client defines as his or her problem. I have come to believe that feelings create thoughts, feelings change feelings, and this dynamic can be used in therapy."

Psychotherapy Theory on Emotions from Freud to Greenberg

Until I began writing this book, I had never heard of anyone who seriously proposed this simple notion. Turns out Spinoza said something similar in the seventeenth century. He said, "An emotion cannot be removed unless opposed or replaced by a stronger one" (Spinoza, 1982, p. 195). Other than Spinoza, no serious thinker prior to Greenberg and his colleagues have entertained the thought that emotions change emotions.

The theory of psychotherapy's emphasis on undoing repression is so well traveled that most psychotherapy students and practitioners can repeat it in great detail. It is difficult to imagine that no serious thinker—from Freud (1935, 1936) to Jung (1946, 1953) to Reich (1942, 1949) to Dollard and Miller (1950) to Rogers (1954) to Perls (1947) to Polster and Polster (1973) to Janov (1970) to Mahrer (1978)—understood that each emotion had its own distinct dynamic and that this fact might provide openings for emotional and characterological change.

Freud (1935, 1936) talked about emotions as if they were one thing. If there was one emotion that captured therapists' attention before Greenberg, it was anxiety or fear. That was Freud's main emotional construct. Behaviorists like Wolpe and Rachman (1960), and Stampfl (1967) inherited their focus on anxiety from Freud. It wasn't until Bandura (1973) that psychotherapists began to consider anger and aggression as a focus of treatment. Bandura's answer to aggression seemed to be to stop watching television and to choose more passive players and mentors as models for behavior. Bandura's modeling theory had very little to do with psychotherapy.

The first real therapeutic recognition of an emotion beyond fear and fear-based sadness was a cognitive behavioral treatment of anger espoused by Novaco (1997). He seemed to be the first clinical theorist concerned about anger. Cognitive behaviorists espoused an intervention called "thought stopping." The technique is simple. Attach a rubber band to your wrist. When you feel inappropriate anger, snap the rubber band against your wrist, thus negatively reinforcing anger.

Many authors, Greenberg and myself included, think that this is a rather silly intervention. Many believe the unconscious doesn't register the negative. Attending to anger by telling one's self not to feel this way only perpetuates the feeling. It does not work to tell someone not to feel what they feel.

Prior to Greenberg (1987, 1991, 1997, 2001, 2002), Gendlin (1996) suggested that each emotion should be explored and used in psychotherapy, but Gendlin did not suggest how to use each emotion. Greenberg coined the term "Emotion-Focused Therapy" with a book by the same name *Emotion-Focused Therapy: Coaching Clients to Work Through Their Feelings*. But again Greenberg doesn't seem to actually do anything in psychotherapy that is different from a Gendlin/Rogerian empathic treatment. He encouraged therapists to use the therapeutic encounter to provoke feelings in the session and to transform feelings with therapeutic attention. This strikes me as very similar to what Carkhuff (1969) calls "immediacy," meaning to focus on the feelings occurring in the moment. Most would recognize this approach to be good therapeutic work, but I'm not sure it is anything really new.

What I am proposing is that therapists teach clients the emotional dynamics of the feelings they are struggling with. The therapist and the client then collaborate to develop a ritual that the client might use several times each day to develop a broader emotional range and to create new emotional paths. The client practices this ritual between sessions to help expand his or her emotional range.

Psychotherapy and Religion

A few years ago, I visited a grand cathedral in Como, Italy. I was walking and looking, oohing and aahing in the hopes of placating my wife, when I first realized that much of what we do in psychotherapy has been stolen from religion. My back was complaining, telling me that I could walk and look no more. I discovered several rows of chairs.

As I sat down in the back row, I observed a line of people waiting their turn to kneel before a priest. This was an open confessional. The priest sat on a raised platform where everyone could see him. As it became their turn, each person walked forward, knelt before the priest, and spoke softly to him for a moment. I presumed they said, "Forgive me, Father, for I have sinned," and then confessed some sin. The priest listened, read something to the parishioner, then looked at the parishioner and spoke directly. I presumed he said something like, "You are forgiven. Say ten Hail Marys. Go forth and sin no more." The person then walked over to sit in one of the chairs, where she contemplated, knelt and prayed in front of a cross, made the sign of the cross, and left.

Here is why I say that what the priest did was much like what I do. If I were to design a healthy intervention for an untrained person to perform with people coming to them for help, it would be something like this. The person would come to the priest. The priest would listen as the individual unburdened herself, and she would leave, having been forgiven. I hope that today's psychotherapists have more to offer than ten Hail Marys and some moralisms. But how different is this from Rogerian psychotherapy?

Our behaviorist forbearers have borrowed a great deal of what they do from the Hindu practice of meditation. Mesmer went to India to learn about

Indian medicine. Instead of learning what the yogi master believed was most important (the self-mastery of emotions), Mesmer brought back hypnosis to the West, not as a tool of self-mastery, but as a tool to control others. This seemed silly to the Hindus.

Psychologists took this hypnosis protocol and taught clients to use it for themselves. They called their intervention systematic desensitization, but it is more or less the same as basic mediation. Every major religion has some version of chanting and meditation as an important spiritual discipline.

The sermon, or homily in the Islam, Judeo-Christian tradition, is a version of cognitive behavioral therapy; it tells people how to think. A visit to one's rabbi, mullah, priest, or minister for consultation in the faith is also a version of cognitive behavioral therapy.

Zen practice with a Zen master has a great deal in common with psychoanalysis. Tavistock-styled group therapy is often called Zen practice in a group setting, because of the collective frustrations it creates in a group.

What I have borrowed from religion is prayer, not exactly prayer to a god, but a ritual repeated several times a day. My mother began everyday with religious readings and prayer. When her children were grown, she continued to use 30 minutes of her day in this religious practice, followed by 30 minutes of physical exercise. The purpose for her daily prayer was to prepare her spirit for the day, to give her mind and heart a cleansing so that she could open herself to her God and to people with a healthy, loving spirit.

This is very similar to what I am proposing we teach our clients. Many faiths have prayer rituals. Muslims turn to Mecca five times daily in prayer. Catholics ritualistically pray, using rosary beads. Many people meditate and consult the I-Ching like my mother used her Bible readings and prayer. The point of this practice according to one such practitioner is "to do something to my brain. I hope that somehow the I-Ching will allow me to be a more aware, conscious, and whole person in the day I'm about to be a part of."

I propose to use what we know about emotions to build a ritual with our clients to give them something that they can do daily to become a more emotionally healthy and balanced person.

Cognitive Behavior Theory Revisited

After I explained this to my colleagues in my consultation group, Tom said, "I get it. That's why this works. One emotion resolves or changes another emotion through chemistry. You are proposing that people can wash their own brains."

"Oh my god, David," Jane said. "You are brainwashing, using our own natural brain chemicals."

"That's right," I replied. "And turning off and on different brain circuits that are associated with different emotions. And people can practice changing their own brain chemicals and their emotions. Basic emotions aren't new, but applying them therapeutically is a new idea."

"That's what makes this a good idea," Tom added. "It's obvious. It's common sense. That's David's contribution. He did that in his sense of community theory.[1] He puts a template on chaos, and it becomes obvious. He has done it again."

"What I like about this," Ralph said, "is that this can be a daily practice.

"Psychoanalysis suggests that deep, real change can only occur over time and with lots of work. Since managed care won't support analytic work, clients can use these rituals. Emotional rituals practiced daily will create cognitive dissonance. Clients will have so much time and energy invested that they will change simply because of the investment. Anything practiced over time and guided by a therapist can bring real change and new emotional postures."

"Much like psychoanalysis," Tom said, "except not as expensive."

"You like that word 'postures' don't you, Ralph?" Jane interjected, trying to distract Ralph from Tom's dig. "I heard you use it in what you just said."

"Yes," Ralph said. "It's better than the psychoanalytic term 'defenses.' I think we all should be grounded in the various ways we create impressions. The descriptions of these 'defenses' in the psychoanalytic literature offer a variety of tools for any therapist. Nancy McWilliams has written the most readable explanation of these defenses. Like Freud, she sees defenses as attempts to protect us from our fears. Fear, for her, is the motivation for engaging a defense. I use the word 'posture' to mean more or less the same thing, our way of posing to create an impression. This may serve to protect us from our fears, as Freud suggests, or it may be used proactively as a resource or tool that helps us reach a goal. The term 'posture' does not have the negative connotation of the term 'defense.'"

"And I think each emotion is a posture," I said. "An emotion may serve to protect and defend, or it can help us communicate, cajole, and organize. An emotion is a tool that can have many purposes. I agree with you, Ralph. The word 'defenses' is too limiting."

"I want to change the subject," said Tom. "David, tell me how this is different from cognitive behavioral therapy. I get it that your approach helps people feel better, while cognitive behavioral therapy helps people think better. But is that it?"

"No," I said, "but before we decimate the easy target of cognitive behavioral therapy, I think we should give the devil his due. Cognitive behavioral therapy gave us something that therapists might do effectively in the short amount of time managed care allowed. It focused on expecting therapy to produce change in behavior. It took the emphasis on the therapeutic bond and shifted it to the work the client was willing to do to get better. This de-emphasized the importance of the therapist and the therapeutic session and emphasized homework and practice that clients did on their own, outside the therapy hour."

"We therapists have a tendency to think it is all about us and the therapy relationship, don't we?" Tom commented.

"And sometimes it is," Jane said, coming to Ralph's defense, in hopes that he would ignore Tom's challenge, and he did.

"Okay, so that's what's good about cognitive behavioral therapy," Ralph said. "What's the dark side?"

"Cognitive behavioral therapy has as a premise that beliefs or cognitive distortions are the cause of dysfunction," I replied. "I think, along with Greenberg and his colleagues, that distorted beliefs are the result of dysfunction, not the cause. Reason does not rule passion. Feelings generate thoughts. Changes in thinking come from changes in feeling. I'm not sure that one can transform rage with the snap of a rubber band on the wrist. I'm not sure real lasting change will come from a cognitive self-lecture that tells us not to feel this way."

"Here, here!" Tom said.

"Amen, Hallelujah," Ralph agreed.

"But David, you are proposing things that are very similar to the cognitive behavioral therapists," Jane said. "Clients can use your ritual like a manualized treatment. You will probably teach skills and some clients will be offended. They will accuse you of treating them with a book, just as we do now with cognitive behavioral therapists."

"Yes," I agreed. "This approach is definitely aimed at emotional skill building."

"Yes, and many clients want a relationship that makes them feel safe," Ralph said. "They have had enough of people trying to teach them and change them. They need a place where they are safe to be."

"I agree," I said. "That is the limiting part of this therapy. It is for people who want information and who want homework. It is not for the many clients who need our love and attention more than they need information."

The group then went on to inquire about the emotion theory that I used to develop my rituals.

The Journey to Tomkins's Emotion Theory

The history of philosophy and psychology is filled with debates over which is superior, reason or emotion. The debate smacks of a couple's argument that we, as couples' therapists, see daily in our offices. One can just hear one member of the couple saying, "My feelings should matter," while the other counters, "Why can't you just listen to reason?" We therapists understand that often reason is a defense against expressing feelings. The same appears to be true of philosophers in this debate. Plato 427–347 B.C. (1974) and Aristotle 384–322 B.C. (1941) thought that emotion was the antithesis of reason. Reason, they believed, was a good thing. Emotion they saw as bad, mysterious, and uncontrollable. Descartes was the first philosopher to take exception to this. Though he took a less defensive approach to emotions, he was the same philosopher who formalized mind/body dualism that psychologists have been trying to undo for some time.

One can be more sympathetic to Descartes's mind/body dualism when his ideas are put in the context of the times. He was attempting to take on the Church, using the mind as a tool against superstition. Incidental to his argument against superstition was his contention that emotions were the place where the mind and the body met. Descartes identified six basic emotions: wonder, fear, love, hatred, joy, and sadness. He saw these emotions as positive human resources.

After Descartes, emotions continued to be a philosophical ping-pong ball pitted against reason. Spinoza (1982) thought emotions were bad. Hume (1739) said some were good. Kant (1953b) said they were bad because emotions disrupted reason. Nietzsche (1967) thought they were good, saying emotions had more reason than did reason itself. In the twentieth century, philosophy abandoned emotion to psychology, becoming interested in the science/faith debate instead.

Psychology demonstrated the same ambivalence toward emotions, as did philosophy. Darwin did a good job starting off the scientific inquiry into emotions in 1872. He named 16 basic emotions. For Darwin, emotions were not opposed to reason. Each emotion had a species-adaptive purpose. They were survival tools. He saw emotions as neurologically wired instincts that originated in the body, primarily the face. (His ideas later greatly influenced my hero emotion theorist, Sylvan Tomkins.)

In the mid-1880s, James (1884) and Lange (1885) independently and simultaneously came upon the same idea. This idea united the mind and body, as did Darwin's thesis. They claimed that we feel emotion before we are aware of what we are feeling. In other words, emotion precedes cognition. (This is the basis of Greenberg's critique of cognitive behavioral therapy.)

After James and Lange, psychology's treatment of emotion became behaviorist dogma. Watson (1924) and his black-box theory contended that, except for fear (à la Freud), we had no hardwired, instinctive emotions. All emotions were learned. The cognitive approach to emotions was extended through Cannon (1927), who vehemently attacked the James/Lange theory. This cognitive approach continues to have its supporters (Ellsworth, 1994;

Chwalisz, Diener, & Gallagher, 1988; see reviews by Cahill, 1996; Demaree & Harrison 1997; Cacioppo, 2000). These theorists all espouse some version of Canon's criticism of James/Lange, which is that we are aware of what we feel before we express it.

In addition to opposing James and Lange, the behaviorists were attacking Freud and his notion of the unconscious. Freud (1935) suggested that one force organized human behavior. That force was the libido. The libido was the desire to live, exist, survive, and procreate. (Much of the literature that focuses on the libido often overemphasizes the procreate part of Freud's notion of libido [Rilling, 2000].) For Freud, the libido organized emotion into two kinds: positive emotions, which are the result of satisfying libidinal urges, and negative emotions, which are the consequence of frustrating the libidinal drives.

This was more or less the state of the debate about emotions around the time that Sylvan Tomkins (the hero of our story) went on sabbatical in the 1940s (Nathanson, 1992). Like many other male academic psychologists, he scheduled his sabbaticals about the time that his wife was to give birth. And, like many brilliant psychological theorists before him, the fascination with his child combined with his thinking about psychological phenomena. I would bet that he couldn't take his eyes from his child's face. While looking at his child, as a father, he also saw her face as if he were Darwin discovering affect in evolutionary theory.

Tomkins's first theoretical observation of his child was powerful. In 1981, he posited that a newborn infant does not know why it cries—it merely cries. Tomkins further theorized that emotions are hardwired, genetically transmitted mechanisms that are universal to humans and animals.

Tomkins began to examine an infant's facial expressions. He proposed that the face was the seat of emotions, that emotions were expressed in the face and perceived by our minds after they formed on our face. This notion united Darwin and James/Lange and extended their theories. Tomkins's study of an infant's facial expressions produced nine specific basic emotions: interest/excitement, enjoyment/joy, surprise/startle, fear/terror, distress/anguish (or sadness/grief), anger/rage, dissmell,[2] disgust, and shame/humiliation.

Writing in 1981, Tomkins said emotions worked as a species survival tool in this way: they amplify and organize the body's response to the stimulus that set them in motion. "Affect makes good things better and bad things worse" (Nathanson, 1992, p. 57). Emotions unite behavior, cognition, and physiology.

According to Tomkins, it was arbitrary to separate these three domains. "Affect causes behavior all over the body" (Nathanson 1992, p. 60). Each domain influences the other. Affect can precipitate cognition, and cognition can precipitate affect. Emotion directs our attention and provides the depth and color for our memory. The autonomic nervous system (ANS) can have little to do with creating an emotion, or it can have everything to do with initiating the affective processes. The muscles in the face are as important to affective experience as the gray matter in the brain. As the face expresses a feeling, the autonomic nervous system correlates to facial expression; cognitive awareness of the feeling follows. And the brain uses genetically determined neurological circuitry with each specific emotion (Davidson, Ekman, Saron, & Senulis, 1990). Tomkins introduced this idea of a central-assembly system, a place in the brain responsible for the focus and maintenance of attention and recruitment of appropriate affect.

While embracing Tomkins's theory, many recent theorists using neurological research discount the face as the emotion center (Buck, 1999). Current emotion theorists do not believe that the face expresses emotion as a separate bodily function, amplifying other mechanisms of behavior to support the basic emotion expressed by the face. Drives such as sex, thirst, and hunger can have their own specific neurological motivational circuitry that might include and express affect but are not created by affect.

"The point on which there is a consensus around Tomkins," writes Buck (1999), "is that affects can constitute primary innate biological motivating mechanisms that can be engaged by other systems" (p. 302). Tomkins is particularly useful when we draw on his specific emotions to understand higher level cognitive, social, and moral behavior.

Paul Ekman is today's anointed son of Tomkins. More than any other, he has researched and extended Tomkins's theory. Cal Izard is also such a candidate. The problem with Izard is that he has to some extent appropriated Tomkins' theory as his own (Nathanson, 1992). Izard's writing and work, however, have more relevance to clinical practice than do those of any heirs of the Tomkins tradition. Perhaps that is because Izard was also a practicing therapist.

Ekman and Izard both set out to prove that Tomkins had indeed discovered the nine basic human emotions. They conducted cross-cultural studies using categorizations of human facial expression. A series of studies have been conducted in this way. In 1971, Izard claimed to have found eleven essential emotions, while in 1994 Ekman claims to have found seven. Ekman, however, is open to others being confirmed later.

Both Ekman and Izard report cross-cultural studies that demonstrate that Darwin and Tomkins are correct. Human facial expressions are interpreted universally the same way. They conducted studies in Japan, Argentina, Chile, and Brazil, but the most convincing studies were conducted in the Highlands of Papua New Guinea, among people who were so isolated that they had never seen movies or pictures interpreting emotions. In all the experiments, people from every culture interpreted the pictures in the same way.

Space does not allow a review of these studies (see Keltner & Ekman, 1996). Suffice it to say that after much criticism and seeming relentless attacks, these studies have basically withstood their assaults. There is wide agreement on Ekman's seven basic emotions and some debate on whether or not to add others.

Another line of research has used the Tomkins 1962 model to discover emotion markers in the autonomic nervous system. Ekman and his colleagues lead the field here as well. Ekman, Friesen, and Levenson have published several articles with different author arrangements and different documented dates (1983, 1990, 1991, 1992) for discovering sets of anatomical markers of specific emotions. Stemmler (1989), Boiten (1996), Sinha and Parsons (1996), and Miller and Wood (1997) are just a few of the other scientists who have recorded specific ANS correlates to specific emotions (see Cacioppo, Tassinary, & Fridlund, 1990, for a review).

Other researchers have focused on neurological substrates in the brain and specific neurohormones that are active during the expression of emotion. The invention of magnetic imaging has done a great deal to aid this endeavor. Panksepp (1991) and his colleagues have done great work in this field. Panksepp irritatingly renames the emotions as if he discovered them. But his writing is clear and his research excellent. Davidson is the leader in the Ekman camp of researchers discovering the emotion brain circuitry. Studies using MRI have found a great deal of hardwired emotional neurocircuitry, and neurochemists have identified a number of neurohormones active in specific emotions (Davidson, 1993).

What Ekman, Frierson, Levenson, and Davidson collectively discovered was when certain facial muscles were engaged, this stimulated reciprocal neurocircuits and neurohormones. This means that emotions work from outside in as well as from inside out. Expressing a feeling in the face will create the internal neurological experience of that emotion. It is also true that imagining or remembering a feeling will stimulate the neurological and facial expression of that feeling. The ability to choose one's own emotional experience by imagining, remembering, and facially expressing a chosen feeling is the skill we hope to promote to purposefully change our own neurochemistry.

Emotion theory debate was especially rancorous and even vicious in the last part of the twentieth century (but perhaps that has always been the nature of the debate on emotion). In fact, discussion has become so extreme that the National Advisory Council was formed by the National Advisory Mental Health Council, Rockville, Maryland, to help clear the air and to focus responsible debate and research. Members began by stating a consensus of what was known about emotions at that time (1995). Without giving a nod to a single emotion theorist, the Advisory Council confirmed Tomkins's basic theory. They wrote in *The American Psychologist* (1995; vol. 50, p. 839):

Our maturing scientific perspective on emotion owes much to the recent explosion of technology that has permitted researchers to describe and measure aspects of emotional life in unprecedented richness and detail. Using sophisticated monitors, behavioral scientists can now tract respiration, heart rate, muscle contractions, facial expressions, voice changes, brain activity, and other objectively measurable aspects of emotion.—Researchers now use these and other emerging technologies to bring rational understanding to emotion, an aspect of behavior long regarded as irrational.

They confirmed the existence of cross-cultural agreement on Ekman's seven basic emotions. They reported evidence for three emotions that exist at birth: surprise, distress (or fear), and pleasure (or joy). By the age of 4 months, a child's anger, too, is clearly visible. By 6 months, shyness and fear appear. Later, complex emotional responses such as guilt/shame, empathy, and pride become a part of the child's emotional repertoire, according to the Council.

At this point (1995), the Council said that science has matured to the place where we now know something about emotions. This is a good jumping-off place to develop a theory of emotions that will be useful in psychotherapy. I believe such a theory can explain and unite much of the theories used in clinical practice to date. The only surprising element about this simple notion is: Why have not discrete emotions and their movement from one to another been a central focus of psychotherapy theory and practice before now?

My Basic Emotions and Why

My consultation group continued its discussion.

"What are your basic emotions?" Tom asked.

"They are fear, anger, sadness, joy, surprise, disgust, shame, interest/desire, and fatigue/rest/trance/sleep," I said.

"Why these?" Jane wondered.

"I used six of Ekman's seven basic emotions. They are: fear, anger, sadness, joy, surprise, and disgust. Ekman has both contempt and disgust. For clinical purposes, these two can be treated as the same emotion."

"So how did you choose your other three?" Jane asked.

"What are they again?" Tom asked.

"They are shame, interest, fatigue/rest/sleep/trance," I answered.

"Before you explain that, what about the terms affect, emotion, and feelings?" Tom wondered. "Many emotion theorists contend these words have different meanings."

"For me, and I think for most clinicians, the distinctions among these terms become pedantic and unnecessary. So, in my book, they all mean the same," I explained.

"So, how did you choose your other three basic emotions?" Ralph asked.

"Well, is shame a hard sell to therapists?" I countered.

"No," Jane said. "That's a basic human emotion."

"Yes," Tom said. "It's in my office with every client."

"Agreed," Ralph concurred. "Why did Ekman leave shame off his list?"

"Ekman has eight criteria in considering whether an emotion should be considered a basic emotion," I answered. "One is that the emotion be present at birth or soon after and have its own physiology. Shame might be a complex emotion that includes fear and sadness, rather than a single emotion, and it is not present at birth, or soon after. It develops later as the brain develops. Ekman suggested that further research might indeed identify shame and other emotions beyond his seven as also basic human emotions, but that right now the data does not support including shame. Of course, we all would agree to include shame."

"Yes," they said in one voice.

"But David, what about guilt?" Jane asked.

"Yeah," Ralph said. "These are two different emotions. I forget which is which. One is what others impose on you about something you did, and the other is what you impose on yourself—it's about the core of who you are."

"Guilt," Tom said, "is about something you did. Shame is about who you are."

"I'm not sure that our clients make that fine distinction," I replied. "I think that is a more recent definition imposed on the therapy world. But the general public, like Ralph, either gets them confused or sees them as one and the same."

"Yeah, I think that's right," Jane said. "I confuse them too."

"The emotions I chose are ones that you can recognize when you see them on someone's face," I said. "That is an important criteria that Ekman imposes as well. And there is no expressive difference between guilt and shame. I treat them as the same basic emotion. Make sense?"

"Yes," they agreed.

"The next emotion," I continued, "is one that I think will also be an easy sell to therapists."

"Which one is that?" Jane asked.

"Interest/desire/excitement," I explained. "I use these three words to represent this emotion to illustrate the problem it presents to the academics. This emotion is not on or off. It has a modulating function like a volume control. This is too confusing for researchers."

"Yes," Tom said. "Researchers don't easily tolerate dimensions in variables."

"I contend," I said, "that our pantheon of emotions should include some emotion that represents motivating forces, for example, appetites like sex, hunger, greed, power, and fame. Many emotion researchers include this emotion as a basic emotion. Using all three words—interest/desire/excitement—represents the range of this emotion from low to medium to high and symbolizes the fact that this emotion has this kind of movement."

"This is Freud's libido," Ralph said. "It makes sense to include this one to me."

"I think we need to include an affective drive system. This makes sense to me too," Tom added.

"Me, too," Jane said. "What I want to see is how you can include fatigue/rest/sleep and the trance."

"This emotion is what interest/desire/excitement is not," I said. "Sleep is to emotions as zero is to numbers. When considering numbers, we might ignore zero because it has no value. But zero is as important a number as one, two, or nine. To ignore sleep as a basic emotion is as similar an oversight as ignoring zero in numbers. I believe the at-rest state is as much a basic part of the human experience as joy, fear, or sadness."

"But what about Ekman's eight criteria?" Tom wondered. "How does this match up to them?"

I began to list them. "They are: (1) automatic appraisal; (2) common antecedents; (3) presence in other primates; (4) quick onset; (5) temporary duration; (6) unbidden occurrence; (7) distinctive physiology; and (8) characteristic display.

"Regarding criterion 1, automatic appraisal, isn't it obvious to any observer when someone's asleep, tired, or bored, or in a trance? Clearly, there are common antecedents—criterion 2—which precede sleep. Exhaustion and lack of stimulation are probably the two most obvious. Of course, sleep is present in other primates. That takes care of criterion 3.

"Can sleep have a quick onset? Criterion 4. Of course, sometimes it does. Don't you know of people with narcolepsy or people who have been so exhausted that they fell asleep in their plate while eating or even in mid-sentence?

"Criterion 5, temporary duration, depends on what 'temporary' means. Sleep can be as short as 1 minute or even a few seconds. It can easily last up to 10 or 12 hours. Criterion 6 is unbidden occurrence. Certainly, children prove each day that they get tired and go to sleep even when they don't want to. Criterion 7, does sleep have its own distinctive physiology? Yes. According to Cantero,[3] five different brain waves are exhibited during sleep. The whole body participates in sleep.

"Criterion 8 is characteristic display. Surely, eyes closed, mouth relaxed, fingers slightly curled, rapid-eye movement, low heart rate are clear signs of sleep."

"How can you have all these words representing this one emotion?" Jane asked.

"As I said," I responded, "this emotion is the antithesis of interest/desire/ excitement. Just as it has dimensions, so does fatigue/rest/sleep/trance. It moves from a hunger for rest or fatigue, to rest, to trance, and then to sleep."

"And, if you are going to say every emotion has a healthy resolve," Tom questioned, "what are you going to use to resolve fear if you leave out this emotion? We use the relaxation response or the trance to treat phobias and panic attacks all the time."

"How would you explain EMDR [Eye Movement Desensitization and Reprocessing] without the trance?" Jane asked.

"I agree," Ralph said.

"Me, too," added Tom. "So you've sold us on your basic nine emotions. But I have a problem with having just nine emotions. What about emotions we encounter every day in therapy sessions with our clients, emotions like anguish, dread, anxiety, disappointment, love, pleasure, or wicked feelings like hate, envy, greed, and so forth?"

"Some of them, like disappointment or anxiety, are just other words for the basic emotions, sadness and fear," I said. "Others are complex emotions. For example, anguish is a combination of fear, anger, and sadness; envy is a combination of desire, sadness, and anger. In reality, emotions are rarely felt as a pure entity without other emotions mixed in. But I can't explain the theory focusing first on the real world."

"Ambiguity is the truth," Ralph said. "Clarity is a distortion of the truth. David, as he always does, speaks to clarify, hence to distort."

"Yes, I suppose," I agreed, "but even in the mixture of emotions often there are healthy and pathological combinations, and often one emotion is the dominant emotion in the mix."

"R. D. Laing called this complex of pathological emotions, 'knots,'" Tom said. "The concept of knots takes advantage of David's idea that emotions resolve into each other. This can create a pathological emotional cycle or knot. These emotions might consist of two emotions bouncing back and forth between one another, or a repeating cycle of three or more emotions. The most common, well-known knots are the depression knots. There are three of them. One resolves sadness with anger. In anger, the person does something stupid, which creates shame, which is resolved by sadness and so on (sadness, anger, shame, sadness). The other depression knot resolves sadness with fear, which feels, to the person, like cowardice, and becomes shame, which is resolved by sadness and so on (sadness fear shame sadness). The third knot begins with interest/desire and is followed by fear of failure, which is followed by letting go of the interest, which is sadness, which is resolved by interest/desire (interest, fear, sadness, interest). When it becomes too dangerous to access interest/desire, we are left with fear and sadness."

"Cal Izard, remember him?" I said. "He taught at Vanderbilt and introduced me to emotion theory. He has described what he called the hostility triad. Rozin called it the CAD complex. This is just a knot using anger to achieve a goal. Once the goal is achieved, joy follows, and, after joy, comes disgust at one's adversary."

"That's a pretty mean, disgusting knot," Jane said.

"Yes, it is. I imagine there are as many pathological knots as there are combinations of various emotions. But you are right, Ralph. My job here is not to describe reality's confusion. It is to tease apart the elements of our emotional experience and help us understand them and master them."

"I would like to get back to your theory," Tom said. "The thing I don't like about the lineage of your theory is this: If you combine mind and body as Darwin, James, Lange, Tomkins, Ekman, Izard, Greenberg, and you do, you will always be the victim of your emotions. We need a theory that helps us master our feelings and one that at the same time conceptualizes the unity of the body and mind."

"That's what David is trying to do here," Ralph said.

"Is that right?" Jane asked.

"Yes, I think it is, now that Tom has put it in these terms. I am trying to recognize that we do feel before we think; that emotions can come on us, as if out of nowhere. Yet, I want to use this reality as a tool we can use to create, so that we are not just subject to our feelings as if they were a disease that we catch. Yes, I think feelings are contagious. But I also believe we can choose to bring to ourselves the next feeling. We can master our attention—and we can use our imagination and memories to create fantasies that bring with them a certain new emotion that will bring with it a healthy resolve of the old emotion."

"I get it," Tom said. "We cannot avoid the reality that emotion precedes cognition, but that does not mean we have to become victims of our feelings. It is because our bodies and minds are one unit that we can focus our minds on a new feeling and that feeling will come."

"This sounds cognitive behavioral to me," Jane said.

"I'm not telling clients what thoughts to think," I said. "I am only asking them to remember or imagine a scene that contained the feeling that they want to feel next, a feeling that will lead them to a healthy constructive resolve out of their stuck emotional place."

"David's theory assumes, as I do," Ralph said, "that feeling one emotion all the time is sickness. Health is an emotional balance, where we flow naturally through all our emotions."

"So," Jane said, "I'm still not clear on how we can use this idea that emotions resolve one another and that we can use emotions, rather than thoughts, to free us from an unhealthy emotional hole or knot."

"I think we are all predisposed to expressing some emotions while avoiding others," I said. "When we know which emotions we allow ourselves to feel and which ones we avoid, we know where we need to work. We are often stuck in the emotions we feel most easily. We need to use the emotions we avoid to help us change our emotional habits."

"Why do you think we tend toward some emotions and avoid others?" Tom asked.

"Our families taught us," Ralph answered.

"Perhaps," I said, "or perhaps we were born this way. I don't think the reason matters. What matters is that we need to find a way to become comfortable expressing all our feelings. There is a time to every purpose."

"The Birds," Jane said.

"Peter, Paul, and Mary before them," I added.

"Who are the Birds and Peter, Paul, and Mary?" Tom wondered.

"Seventies' rockers and sixties' folk singers. They sang those words."

"The words come form the Old Testament, Ecclesiastes 3:1," Ralph explained. "They make David's point. There is a purpose for each emotion, and, to be a whole, healthy person, we need to feel all of them. Most of us feel the ones we want to feel and avoid the others. David's right."

"So, how do we use this in therapy?" Jane asked.

"Well, in the therapy hour, you can help your clients know which emotions they need to work on," I said. "You can model for them and teach them how to move out of an emotionally stuck place and back into the natural emotional flow that can include all their feelings. And between sessions, you can give them rituals they can use to become masters of their emotional process."

"But to do that," Ralph said. "We must know how emotions work and which ones work best to resolve unhealthy emotional knots and patterns."

"This is an interesting theory," Jane said. "I would trust it more if I understood how you came to this."

How I Came to This

The answer to that question was too complicated for me to answer there. In 1971, I took an emotions course from Cal Izard and read his book, *The Face of Emotion* (1971). Later, I read Donald Nathanson's book *Shame and Pride* (1992). These books introduced me to Sylvan Tomkins (1962, 1963, 1981), but these things had little to do with my ability to understand this theory. I was only 25 when I first read about Tomkins. I had not yet seen my first client.

The First Time

This idea first occurred to me 15 years later on my wedding day. I have always teared-up at weddings, and I was especially concerned that I might fall apart at my own. I was determined to keep my composure and speak audibly in declaring my commitment to my bride, Marietta.

The guests were gathered. The photographer had begun taking pictures (and sipping the wine). Marietta's father, a minister, was to perform the service. He specifically instructed the photographer not to take pictures during the ceremony, because he wanted no distractions from this important moment. I sensed the photographer wasn't paying attention to his admonitions. I asked a friend to keep an eye on her to make sure she was not shooting during the ceremony.

The ceremony began. I was standing before my future father-in-law, Marietta at my side, all of us in front of a large picture window. We were nearing the part where I would have to say something. Emotions began to flood over me. Tears filled my eyes. I was choking. I wasn't sure I would be able to speak.

The momentum of this sad joy seemed beyond my control, until I saw the photographer tiptoeing outside the house and behind the large picture window. Anger poured into my body. I motioned to my friend to go outside and rein her in. He moved immediately. Marietta's father turned to me cueing me to speak. "I do" I spoke with a clear, strong voice. The flow of the sad, tearful hormones had been replaced in an instant by angry neurohormones. My composure returned, and I was able to perform as I had hoped, thanks to the photographer and my anger.

Since that day, I wondered if somehow I could use this same physiological law (anger resolving sadness) with my clients. Sometimes, when I saw a depressed client, I would think, "I wish he would just get mad." I would dismiss that thought and do what I had been trained to do: listen carefully; empathize; create a safe, sacred context for the client to find the various parts of himself; integrate them into a new whole; and help him graduate from therapy.

Music and a Metaphor for Feelings

Once I began to open my mind to this way of thinking, ideas began flooding my brain. I kept thinking about music. Emotions are like music. Think about Vivaldi's "Four Seasons." It mirrors moods related to seasonal changes. As I mentioned earlier in this chapter, a musical composition can reflect how emotions work in the brain. We are always feeling something. In a healthy person, that "something" we feel changes, like the shifts in the notes of a symphony. Each musical tone resolves into another. That new note merges with another, and so on. The composer establishes major emotional themes, with undercurrents of other emotions.

Emotions move through us in the same way. This flow can create a brilliantly harmonious symphony, or it can become a discordant hodgepodge. Accomplished composers know which notes to put next to each other to create harmonious melodies. They understand point-counterpoint. They anticipate the effect of major and minor keys upon the listener's emotions.

As I thought about it, emotions could be considered as different instruments played in a symphony. Some instruments are used best in certain parts of a composition. Almost all the instruments could play the notes, but trumpets are best at making announcements. Violins do an excellent job of crying. Tympanies create depth. Some of us try to play all of our emotional music using only one or two instruments. For those folk, therapists should help them learn to play all their instruments so that their emotional symphony has complete expression.

Surely, if we understood emotions as instruments in a symphony orchestra, we could become emotional maestros instead of emotional victims. What if we knew how to purposefully put one emotion next to another to make a harmonious emotional flow? How would this impact our daily lives? Hearing one note, monotonously repeated is comparable to being stuck in one emotion.

Other Metaphors

I saw the same point from another perspective. It is like film in a movie projector stuck on one frame. Eventually, the celluloid frame is overheated by the light bulb, the frame overheats, burns, and the film disintegrates into acrid smoke.

This theory can find another metaphor in color. For some, color is the outward reflection of inner feelings. In literary terms, red is anger, blue represents sadness, and yellow stands for fear. Talented artists create exquisite compositions using harmonious combinations of color. They are masters of knowing which palettes work together to communicate visual beauty. And we all know beauty when we see it. Perhaps we do not understand what we are seeing, but most of the time we agree on what is appealing to the eye.

For instance, two of the most unappealing paintings to a viewer might be a completely black canvas or a blank, white canvas. In emotional terms, this would be equivalent to alexathymia, the expression of no emotion. Why can't we paint with our emotions the way an artist combines colors in a painting?

Wouldn't that be great? If we understood how our emotions work the way artists understand colors, we would be masters of ourselves.

Psychological Mindedness

Then I read John Gottman and colleagues' (1997) famous study of how families communicate emotionally. This was a study of parents who were emotional masters and compared their children with the children of parents who were emotionally ineffective. Gottman followed a cohort of children, ages 4 to 8 years. The experimental subjects were children who had a psychologically emotionally competent parent; the controls did not. The children of the psychologically minded parent scored higher on measures of self-esteem, school performance, sociability, and appropriate behavior. They even scored healthier on measures of vagal nerve tone, as well as general physical health.

Gottman concluded that children with psychologically minded parents are healthier, and more socially capable and intellectually competent, and are more likely to pass on this emotional competence to their children. For clinicians, the point of this study is that if people can become effective at managing their emotions, they can change the quality of their lives and also the lives of those they love.

Changing Emotions Changes Brain Chemistry

My next thought was not so original. Many people are claiming that they can change brain chemistry by changing thought patterns. I'm not sure that changing thoughts will change brain chemicals. But I am sure that changing feelings will change brain chemicals, because chemicals are part of our body's emotional response. We can't change how we feel without changing the brain chemistry.

This is exactly what 14-year-old Portnoy (of *Portnoy's Complaint* [1972]) does. These kids feel embarrassed and ashamed by the awkwardness of their age and their lack of social skills. When they come home from school, they retreat to their rooms, reach between their mattress and box springs, pull out an issue of *Playboy* and imagine they are exactly what they are not. They fill their brain with desire and images of their sexual power, and they change their brain chemistry with masturbatory fantasies.

Girls of the same age often do the same thing with food. They come home from an embarrassing day at school, and they can use food to cover their feelings, or they can purge food as their release. Some girls avoid their painful feelings by starving themselves. Appetite neurohormones, those that accompany a starving person's desire for food, fill their brains. Their hunger and accompanying longings for food cover their unpleasant feelings.

And this is what batterers do after they have been chewed out at work. They come home and cover their shame and fear with rage at their wives and children. These are all drug events, aren't they? Some of us get addicted to these emotions because of the drugs they give us.

Beethoven's Ninth

As I was reflecting on how emotions change emotions one day, I was listening to Beethoven's Ninth Symphony. I heard Beethoven move from fear to anger, to shame, to surprise, to rest, to joy, and back and forth among, what seemed like to me, all nine of the basic emotions. What he did in this piece was amazing, not only musically but emotionally. He found segues between emotions resolving one feeling with another, and that feeling with yet another, until he explored the whole range of human emotions. Listening to this piece in this way, through the frame of this theory, was thrilling.

Wouldn't it be great to have such an emotional range? As a person, I want this kind of mastery for myself. I think if I can begin to understand how Beethoven did what he did in the Ninth Symphony, I can help clients become emotional masters as well.

In this masterpiece, Beethoven gives us the opportunity to use all our feelings. Using all our feelings is the way out of being overly dependent on just a few.

As I further thought about how this theory might affect my practice, another appealing aspect became evident to me. Managed care sometimes forces therapists into unethical boxes. Therapists can no longer treat those patients who need time (lots of it) and our compassion (lots of that, too). So clients come to us, complete with their allotted six to twenty managed-care sessions. When, after twenty sessions, they can no longer afford to see their therapist, they become abandoned once more. They are insulted by the instruction we give them in our new world of cognitive behaviorism. They might fill out the evaluation form, pretending to be helped to gratify the therapist or to conform to what they think others would write. But basically, they have been betrayed once more.

Though I abhor managed care, I must confess that it has forced me to ask myself: What do I have to teach people who come to me, hoping that I have some new information about how they can feel better? Their way of coping with life isn't working. They seem stuck in the same painful emotional cycle. They sincerely want to be taught a new way. They need information. What can I teach them?

My answer is that I can teach them how their emotions work. That's how this theory came to me. That's why I wrote this book.

CHAPTER 2

How Emotions Work
in the Brain and Body

I am proposing that clinicians can use emotion rituals to change emotional patterns, to create new neurological paths, and to employ a broader range of neurochemicals, among other things. For this to be possible, the brain must be able to make use of this disciplined behavior. Several questions about how emotions work in the brain must be answered: Do we feel before we think? Do emotions precede awareness? How does the brain transmit emotional signals? Do our neurochemicals change when our emotions change? Can emotion work with reason? How is the brain designed to enable us to feel and adapt? Why does reason seem to have little effect on emotion?

It is important to note that research on the brain continues at a furious pace—everything is dated once it is written. Neurologist Michael Kaminski recently told me that any current description of how the brain works is soon reduced to a metaphor of how the brain works because of the continuous research and discoveries about the brain. Magnetic resonating imagery now is able to take pictures of brain activity. What were once only theoretical understandings of the brain can be tested and seen.

For us clinicians, this is, perhaps, a useful way to use this information, not as gospel truth, but as an image we keep in our minds as we watch our clients change their emotional patterns and behaviors.

Do Changes in Emotion Change our Brain Chemistry?

Anger is perhaps the most dramatic demonstration of this. Part of the brain is dedicated to determining whether our bodies should be in crisis mode. This is called the amygdala. It is part of the hypothalamus, which is part of the mammalian brain. (Already more than any self-respecting clinician wants to know. More later about the mammalian brain.) If the amygdala determines we are to fight, we feel anger. If it determines we should run, we feel fear.

When the amygdala flips the anger switch, the pituitary gland releases a neurohormone (adrenocortotropic hormone or ACTH, for short) that activates the adrenal glands. The adrenal glands release epinephrine or norepinephrine. These are humoral signals. They communicate to the rest of the body through the bloodstream, giving the signal to dilate the eyes and for the blood to move away from the surface of the skin. This prepares our bodies for wounds and prevents excessive blood loss from injuries. Our pulse rate surges. Our blood vessels constrict. This pumps a lot of blood through our bodies, quickly preparing the body to use its strength.

In a second or less, these chemicals are activated throughout the body. They create a sudden and dramatic change in our bodies and minds. Yes, just as in anger, a change in any emotion changes our brain chemistry. Each emotion has its own set of brain chemicals that it activates and its own neurocircuitry that it uses.

What is a Humoral Signal?

A difference exists between a neurohormone and a neurotransmitter. Neurohormones are humoral signals. These are transmitted through the bloodstream. It is a chemical that acts at a distance from a receptor. Its effects can last a long time, from minutes to hours or days. It amplifies throughout the body. The chemicals used in the humoral system are called neurohormones. The humoral signal initiates the production of proteins all through the body.

To illustrate, let's follow the pituitary gland's release of the neurohormones' ACTH. Once released by the pituitary, ACTH acts on the adrenal gland that releases other neurohormones, epinephrine and norepinephrine, and other steroids. This release of the adrenal neurohormones is sensed by the pituitary, which then stops secreting ACTH. This forms a simple neurohormone feedback loop. Cushing's disease is an example of what happens when this feedback loop is messed up, i.e., the pituitary gland does not turn off. This creates hypercortisolism, which in turns creates obesity, hypertension, diabetes, and labile emotions.

A neurotransmitter is different. It is a chemical, too. For example, serotonin is a neurotransmitter. A neurotransmitter is an ambient fluid in and about the brain and other nerve cells. When the amount of a chemical neurotransmitter builds to a certain level in and around the nerve, the positive to negative chemical balance passes a homeostatic threshold, and the nerve fires. As soon as it fires, the nerve ion balance is restored. It doesn't fire again, unless the brain cells receive more chemicals affecting the positive to negative ion balance.

A neurotransmitter works in conjunction with a nerve cell. Nerve cells are made of a nucleus that is always in balance when its chemical ionic valence is negative. The chemicals outside the nerve center—the neurotransmitters—are positive. The nerves have dendrites or receptor cells. When these cells open and when the positive neurotransmitters are present, the nucleus chemical valence changes from negative to positive. The nerve fires and sends an electrical impulse along what's called an axon. This passes the chemical positive charge along to a nearby nerve cell, which goes through the same process, transmitting the signal throughout the brain and body as an electrical impulse.

As far as therapists are concerned, all we need to understand is that neurotransmitters and neurohormones are chemicals that change when emotions change. The fact that these chemicals work inside two different systems is probably irrelevant to us. In fact, the distinction between the two is blurred in the minds of neuroscientists as well. Dopamine is a neurotransmitter that acts a lot like a neurohormone. In Parkinson's disease, the lack of dopamine can have a humoral effect. The muscles can freeze. The body can become rigid because of the scarcity of dopamine in the brain.

Though most of us don't care whether an emotional change comes from a dendrite, neurohormone, neurotransmitter, or axon, this description of how the brain works provides a consistent picture of what's happening to our clients and to us when they and we feel an emotion.

How Do Emotion and Cognition Work Together?

Emotions work with reason or cognition in several ways. The first is that emotion prioritizes our attention. Reason cannot understand the importance of an event unless we feel an emotion that helps us understand its relevance to us. Without emotion, we cannot know what is best for us to attend to now or next.

Second, if people have a brain injury that involves say, fear, they cannot perceive fear in others or feel fear themselves. Therefore, they often misunderstand others and do not appreciate apparent danger in threatening circumstances. This applies across all emotions. A person's awareness of what's going on suffers if not given the benefit of feeling or expressing that emotion.

Third, emotions are inseparable from the rational ideas of reward and punishment, pleasure or pain, approach or withdrawal, personal advantage and disadvantage. Emotions help us think, but thinking rarely influences how we feel. We are about as effective at stopping an emotion as we are at preventing a sneeze. We can educate our emotions, but not suppress them entirely (Greenberg, 2001).

How Does An Emotion Begin?

It has to do with homeostasis. As something affects either our physical or emotional homeostasis, our emotions are recruited to prepare the body to deal with the change. The emotion recruited depends on the kind of change in our homeostasis. An emotional change will change our physical homeostasis and vice versa.

This means that remembering imagining and thinking will produce an emotion. Consciousness can create feelings. While this is true, reason can only shape our feelings. The controlling power of reason, however, is modest.

How is the Brain Organized?

The brain's architecture is built on our evolution. The first major structure is called the reptilian brain. This is what we share with reptiles. It primarily consists of the brainstem nuclei.

The mammalian brain forms an overlay on top of the brainstem nuclei. This is the second evolution of the brain. It is the part of the brain we share with mammals. Our mammalian brain is about the size of a fist. Most of the neurostructures for our emotions are part of the reptilian and mammalian brains.

The third structure is the additional layer that we humans share. This rather large area, the neocortex, is the source of reason, conscious awareness, and intelligence. This is the part of the brain that rests on top of the mammalian brain, mostly toward the front part of our cranium.

This is why reason has so little effect on emotion. Emotion came first. Emotions create the context for reason. Emotions direct and guide our bodies to the problems we call on our reason and intelligence to solve.

What Controls What?

The parts of our brains that we share with reptiles and mammals are the parts of the brain that control our emotion. Perhaps a mammal could be conscious of an emotion. But could a reptile? Reptiles probably do not perceive or express emotions. Mammals and humans often perceive and express an emotion without being aware of what they are doing. Perception and expression of emotion are independent of awareness. Reason does not control emotion. (In fact, control is too strong a word to use in reference to the brain and emotion. Instead, we should use the word "influence.") The larger human part of the brain, the cerebral cortex lies on top of the brain's emotion center. Hence, we call the area that contains our emotions "subcortical." This includes the brainstem region, the hypothalamus, and the basal forebrain.

Earlier, we discussed how the amygdala controls our vigilance response. While that is true, the brainstem (a part of the reptilian brain) activates most emotions. The brainstem is the part that first responds to a change in our homeostasis. Sadness, as another example (like fear and anger), has its specific neurological circuits. These involve the hypothalamus and ventromedial prefrontal lobe. The other emotions have their own unique emotion centers and wiring as well.

Some parts of the brain connect the cerebral cortex (the brain's newest evolution) to the basal sub-cortex of the emotions (the mammalian brain). The induction sites in the cerebral cortex include parts of the anterior cingulate region and the ventromedial prefrontal region. The body, however, is more connected to emotions through the older parts of the brain (the mammalian brain and the reptilian brain) than it is to the neocortex. (In chapter 4, we will explore each emotion's brain circuitry in more detail.)

Before we studied emotions in psychology, most of us probably assumed that Cannon (1927) was right. Our brains tell us when and what to feel. If true, the cortex would activate emotion. The way the brain is organized makes it clear that this notion is wrong. Reptiles and mammals don't have a cerebral cortex. What turns on an emotion?

Darwin and Tomkins thought emotion originated in the facial muscles. This is a plausible explanation, because the facial muscles and the rest of the emotion system seem to come on all at once. Perhaps emotions do register in our face first and then move through the brainstem, activating the brain chemicals and the neurocircuitry simultaneously.

This explanation, however, ignores the fact that a thought, a memory, or a fantasy can create an emotion. That means that the cortex can create feelings, just as feelings create thoughts in the cortex (Buck, 1988). Emotions can begin internally or externally, either from a thinking event that comes from the neocortex or from an external stimulus that breaks our homeostasis for good or bad. The system can be turned on by internal thoughts, memories, and fantasies, or by external events.

How Do Brain Chemicals Work with the Brain?

Much of the new knowledge about the brain concerns brain chemistry. The brain is not just a bunch of wires going from one emotion center to another. Each emotion center operates different parts of the body to prepare it for action. Emotion brain structures use different neurotransmitters and neurohormones, chemicals that turn on and increase or decrease the amplitude of our emotions. Understanding neurohormones and neurotransmitters and how they work is the Rosetta stone for understanding emotions.

To experience one emotion intensely, the supply of neurotransmitters must be high and the brain receptors in that emotion's brain center must be open. If there is an abundant supply of neurotransmitters and the numbers of receptive brain cells are few, the emotion will not be very intense. If there is a high quantity of an emotion's brain receptors open and a small supply of the emotion's neurotransmitters available, the emotion will not be very intense.

For an emotion to be fully expressed, a high quantity of brain receptors in that emotion's brain centers must be open and an abundant supply of that emotion's neurohormones must be available. That means our emotion's hormones and brain receptors are necessary but not sufficient to feel and express an emotion.

Most of us remember some reference to the limbic system controlling our emotions. Over the years there have been several versions of this system. Some omit parts that other versions include. More recent research has blown the old version of the limbic system to hell (Buck, 1999).

The hippocampus was a centerpiece of the limbic system construct. Now we see it has less to do with emotion and much more to do with memory and information processing. The reason this notion of a limbic system has survived so long is because it included the amygdala. The amygdala, as you recall, is central to the regulation of fear and anger. Though our 1970s version of the limbic system is passé, it is still useful to consider a network of brain parts that are connected to make up the brain's various emotional response centers. What we now know is that the various parts of the brain that serve emotions are not as centrally located as we once thought. We now think the hippocampus gives emotional valence to our memories. It remembers events in order of emotional importance, and it gathers together and organizes memories that are associated with an experience of an emotion. Referring to the emotional part of the brain as the limbic system remains convenient (Buck, 1999), even though not precisely accurate.

How Does the Brain Work in the Body?

There are basically two nerve systems in the body. The first system, of course, is the central nervous system (CNS). This is simply the brain and the spinal cord. The second system extends out from the CNS. That system is called the peripheral nervous system (PNS). This system includes the cranial nerves that connect the facial muscles to the brain, the somatic nerves, connecting the muscles that carry the impulse to move, and the sensory nerves that carry information to the brain about pain, temperature, pressure, and stretch or muscle tension. The autonomic nervous system (ANS) is also part of the PNS. This system is especially relevant to emotions. It helps regulate the body's homeostasis. The hypothalamus is the region of the brain that is connected to the ANS.

The ANS has two parts: the sympathetic system and the parasympathetic system. Together, as the ANS, these two systems control the iris of the eye and the body's lungs, salivary glands, heart, blood vessels, stomach and intestines, sweat glands, liver, spleen, pancreas, bladder, and genitals. Simply put, the sympathetic system are the wires that turn on or contract or initiate secretion in these organs with the exception of the lungs, pancreas, genitals, bladder, and iris of the eye. These organs are relaxed or turned off by the sympathetic system. The parasympathetic system turns on the organs that the sympathetic system turns off. That is why we often confuse them.

The parasympathetic and sympathetic systems are in constant tension with each other, creating the body's organic balance. When one system is dominant, the other system submits. That remains the state of affairs until the once dominant system tires or the other system is stimulated.

This is why this theory works. When we feel one emotion, say anger, this turns on the sympathetic nervous system and turns off the parasympathetic system. When our feelings change to sadness the opposite happens. With sadness the parasympathetic system comes on and the sympathetic system is turned down.

One way to remember which system is which is to associate a vibrant heart with the sympathetic system. The heart needs the lungs to be open, taking in air and feeding oxygen to the blood. The blood vessels need to contract, pushing blood through the body and raising our blood pressure. Sweat glands need to be active to cool the body. You don't need an erection. You need to relax the bladder and tighten its sphincters. The liver needs to push out more glucose, the adrenal gland needs to discharge epinephrine and norepinephrine, and so forth. And when you are asleep or relaxed the opposite happens and the parasympathetic system is dominant.

That's the reason we cannot have sex unless we are relaxed. That's the reason that when fear and sex are associated the result is sexual trauma. And it is the reason consent is essential to healthy sex. It is also the reason Portnoy's masturbation strategy worked to manage shame and fear. Sexual arousal and desire are incompatible with shame and fear.

Summary and Conclusion

At every turn, when we consider the brain's architecture or the ways chemicals work with neurocircuits, the same theme is repeated. Cognition is not central to emotion. But emotion is central to cognition. This means that intuition may have another source of information that does not come from reason or the cerebral cortex.

As you consider the way the sympathetic system collaborates with the parasympathetic system in the ANS, you discover the basis of the famous book *The Relaxation Response* (Benson, 1975). Given that the sympathetic system and parasympathetic system cannot be completely on at the same time, if you turn on one, the other automatically turns off. To combat fear we simply turn on the parasympathetic system. We do this by using abdominal breathing so that our belly moves as we breathe and our chest remains still. We lower our shoulders. We open our hands so that they are not tense. We close our eyes and let our eyes roll back in our heads. We ask our muscles to relax. We empty our mind of thoughts. These actions turn off the sympathetic nervous system, while they turn on the parasympathetic system.

This is, in part, a description of how the emotion rituals work. In the case of *The Relaxation Response*, Benson points out that relaxation replaces fear. This is how we treat phobias. This is the basis of systematic desensitization. And the neurochemicals, the neurohormones, and the neurotransmitters change as the sympathetic dominance is exchanged for parasympathetic dominance. One turns the other off as it comes on and vice versa.

It is not quite so simple for the other emotions. *The Relaxation Response* makes it appear as if, when one system is on, the other is completely off. That is not true. These systems are in constant tension with one another. In a state of moderate alertness, both are moderately on. Rarely is one of these systems so dominant that the other system is completely off. Each emotion has a different amount of homeostatic alertness. Sadness has more parasympathetic dominance. Desire has more sympathetic dominance. The amount of dominance depends on how strong the desire is and so on through all the emotions.

Many of us hate thinking about humans this way. It is reductionistic. We are more than the sum of our parts. Each of us is unique. There seems to be no spirit in this way of thinking.

In response to this, we have to face the reality that we are all more alike than we are different. This, however, does not mean that we aren't different and that each of us is not unique. Some of us have what researchers term "short genes" that give us a predisposition to some emotions over others. We are as similar, I think, as are our taste in food. Though most of us have tastes that overlap, each of us has our own unique appetite.

The point of this description of the brain is not to reduce us to being alike. It is to give therapists another metaphor. Chemicals, interactions, feedback loops, receptors opening and closing—these ideas are descriptions of any system or network made of parts. And in any system fate plays a part; the wind blows. We cannot predict the future. We all have similar but different journeys.

Most importantly from this description of how the brain works (looking at its architecture and how it has evolved), it becomes clear that we cannot think our way out of emotional dysfunction. Our feelings come first. Reason will influence our emotional progressions less than our emotions, because of how the brain is organized. Of course, we have to feel our way to emotional health.

What I do not like about my theory and the rituals that can come from it is that it makes it appear that, as therapists, we are merely technicians. There is a movement in psychology to impose sanctions against therapists who do not use manuals in treatment. What is happening to years of experience and clinical judgment (Levant, 2003)? Some of my ideas smack of the medical model. Diagnose the emotion and give clients a ritual and a pill (Norcross, 2001).

I want to underline some things about this theory that run counter to the notion of manualized treatment. This theory supports intuition. It emphasizes feelings over logic. It questions most of the manualized, cognitive-behavioral-treatment approaches at their foundation. I use science to support therapies that focus on emotions first.

We all know that an effective therapeutic alliance is the best predictor of a positive psychotherapy outcome. We all know that empathy, not a manual, is the primary ingredient to a healthy therapeutic relationship. Clinical judgment about how to care, how to respect, and how to maintain connections and boundaries simultaneously always will be more art than science. My goal is simply to provide the clinician in the field with another tool. And that is all this theory is, one more tool. It is not meant to take the place of or disparage any other theory except for perhaps those of cognitive-behavioral fundamentalists.

My goal in this chapter, and in this book, is to connect science to practice. Making practice conform to science is foolish (Fox, 2003). Practitioners often are ahead of proof (Fox, 2003). Medical doctors were using aspirin before they understood its pharmacodynamics (Olson, 2001). Here, we are trying to build a bridge between common sense and clinical practice. Many of you might have intuited this theory already, but you may not have put it together as I have here. Most clinicians focus on feelings. This book provides a systematic way to understand and use the power of each basic feeling.

Our best work will continue to be based on clinical judgment. Therapy of whatever kind has always depended on the therapist's talent for building a relationship between the therapist and the client. These ideas will never replace that part of our work.

CHAPTER 3

Using Ritual in Psychotherapy

At first, these ideas appeared revolutionary to me. One might imagine a new version of psychotherapy coming from them. A closer look shows that no new therapy is required to accommodate the information presented here. All therapists, using whatever theoretical frame of reference, can use more information about how emotions become linked. Empathy is a therapist's best tool. Empathy is understanding how natural it is for clients to feel as they do. Awareness of emotional patterns and cycles, healthy and unhealthy, make empathy easier. This information without the rituals can be helpful.

Many therapists are immediately repelled by the notion of discipline being a facet of psychotherapy, as was I. But this is not such a new concept. For more than 40 years therapists have been using versions of the CALMS ritual (see chapter 6) in helping clients manage fears. It is part of biofeedback treatment and systematic desensitization, among other treatments aimed toward anxiety and phobias.

Rituals are a useful adjunct to any type of therapy. One important goal of psychotherapy is to empower the client. Too often we therapists believe that the therapist and the therapy are the center of our client's inner life.

Many therapists who interpret dreams often find that the subject of the dreams concerns the psychotherapy relationship itself. Sometimes this interpretation may be true and sometimes it may not. It is often helpful to find emotional dramas inside the psychotherapy relationship, but it does not necessarily empower the client with self-awareness and information about how to cope with the problems of living. Instead, it may merely feeds the therapist's own narcissistic ego.

Rituals help put the growth process more directly in the hands of the client. The work that clients do with rituals belongs to them. Their progress when using a ritual can only be attributed to that individual. Rituals diminish the importance of the therapist and empower the client.

A master therapist, Bob Stepbach, once told this story:

> I saw this boy when he was 13. After testing him, I worked intensely with him and his parents for some months. Years later, I saw him and I recognized him. He must have been in his late twenties. He did not recognize me. It was as if I had never existed. I'm proud of that. That outcome of intervening, helping someone get their life on track, and withdrawing so that you can be forgotten, is the best therapeutic outcome.

Rituals create an opportunity for important work to be done, independent of a therapist. They create a process for growth and healing that depends on the client's energy and commitment to growth. This is a resource to the therapeutic process that empowers the client and gives a tool to the client that can be used throughout life, perhaps instead of returning to the therapist.

Therapists have long been confused by the dichotomy of thinking and feeling. This mind-body duality has plagued occidental thought literally for centuries. Not surprisingly, therapists get caught in this debate as well. Here, this manifests in the debate between humanistic therapies, such as the emotion-focused therapy of Greenberg, and the cognitive-behavioral therapy of Beck. "The resolution to the dilemma of our emotionality vs. reason lies not in privileging one stream of consciousness over the other but in integrating the two" (Greenberg, 2001, p. x). This seems obvious, but if it were simple, it would have been done before now. As long as there are two positions juxtaposed, it is easier to see their differences than to integrate their strengths. Newbrough (1995) suggested that dichotomous thinking creates unnecessary conflict and discord. He suggested a third position be used to mediate the debate between the two.

Greenberg (2001) inadvertently gives an example of how the third position works.

He suggests that toddlers' two-activity schemes of standing on their feet and falling are dynamically synthesized into a higher-level activity scheme for walking. This is a model for how the third position works. Two positions of standing and falling seem to be polar opposites, but patience often brings a third position that demonstrates how all three are interdependent important parts of a whole. The third position in the process of learning to walk, in which standing and falling are part of that process of taking a first step.

Here, the nomination for a third position that seems to shout at us is behavior or action. The experience that functions as the third position and that integrates feelings and thought is action.

Ritual is practice that prepares one for action. Ritual is practiced action that combines thought and feeling. It is directed, purposeful behavior that uses visualization, emotion, and behavior to establish a platform for a successful approach to one of life's problems. Ritual integrates reason, emotion, and behavior. In ritual, we have the head, the heart, and the hands (Langer, 1958).

The human search, beginning with Aristotle (1941) and the "golden mean," was to find a balance between reason and emotion. "But to be angry with the right person, to the right degree, at the right time, for the right purpose, and in the right reason–this is not easy" (Greenberg, 2002, p. 6). This requires practice and more practice. Ritual provides the occasions to practice, integrating our emotions with reason in behavior.

Discipline and Art

Bob Stepbach once told me, "You can't have a quality life unless you are an artist." "I'm not an artist, and I won't ever be," I thought to myself. He went on to explain, and this is the essence of what I remember he said: Each of us has the potential to be an artist. Artists find a medium that they use to annotate and reflect upon life. This requires that the artist take the marginal position of observer, reflector, transformer, and creator. To be an artist requires time alone developing your talent, reflecting on your subject, and transforming your emotions into art.

Most of us spend our time as the hub of a network of people and activity. Many of us see ourselves as the "but-for" person, the essential piece, the key person. The atmosphere of this role, whether real or imagined, is filled with pressure and tension. Quality lives can't be lived in this context. A quality life requires perspective and self-scrutiny. We can't be self-aware when we are the center of attention. Self-awareness comes at life's margins, from the position of the onlooker. When we observe others performing, feeling, and reacting, we see ourselves. When we act as an artist, we use what we learned from the onlooker position in the expression of our art.

While in graduate school, I conducted a study on the quality of life of adolescent 14-year-olds. This was an ecological study that examined the qualities of the various behavior settings that these teenagers inhabited. We interviewed them about their activities on a random day. On the day following the date selected randomly for the study, we interviewed the study participants.

We examined a number of qualities about each setting that they entered. We compared these external variables to a variety of intra-psychic variables, such as self-esteem and general well-being. One of the setting qualities that we focused on was the power level (or what Barker [1968] unfortunately called "the penetration level") that the subject inhabited in each setting. Barker (1968) had six levels of power. Level one was onlooker; level two, guest; three, member; four, active participant; five, co-leader; and six, single leader.

We expected that the more power that our research participant teenagers had the better their scores on the well-being scales. As an afterthought, we examined the variety of levels of each participant, across behavior settings. We found that power did not correlate with general well-being, but that the variety of power levels inhabited by the subjects in their daily settings highly correlated with psychological health. Healthy people need to spend some time at every level of power.

The findings of this study were never published. But they make the same point Stepbach was making: Sometimes people need to get out of the center. They need to spend time at the margins and at all levels of power. Assuming the posture of the artist and using rituals to practice one's art can help give a person perspective and opportunities to reflect.

If we are confined to the producer, key-person roles, we cannot achieve the perspective and distance that we need to examine ourselves, our feelings, and our life experience. Taking on an art form forces us out of the key-person role and gives us a position at the margins, behind a camera, in front of a canvas, with our hands in wet clay, or alone, with pen in hand with a blank sheet of paper. Everyone can express themselves artistically. Everyone has feelings that can be expressed through an art form. To have quality lives, we must find our medium of artistic expression.

So what does art have to do with ritual? Ritual is simply practice of a certain process. That process may be a dance step, a free throw, a golf swing, a turn of a potter's wheel, a mantra or a prayer, or a set of linked, emotional experiences. Ritual is simply about practice and repetition.

Once I studied yoga with an instructor. I had not practiced my yoga all week, and I felt guilty, as I entered her class one evening. I went up to her and confessed. She replied, "What's important is that you have returned to the practice. The ritual of yoga in one's life should be celebrated. Be glad for every stretch and posture you allow yourself to practice. Be thankful that you returned tonight to your practice."

The discipline of an organized practice of any skill is a significant resource for developing that skill. Well-practiced rituals become comfortable and comforting. As rituals are practiced, often we can note improvement. Even if the ritual effectively makes no difference, the placebo effect and the effect of cognitive dissonance will help the ritual become effective, even if there is no other benefit to practice.

It is in the practice that rituals connect to art. Practice is required to develop an artist's talent. If one can accept the discipline of the practice of a ritual, one can become an artist. It takes only a small modicum of talent, dedication to the art form, and practice to master a skill.

Practice rituals in dance are essential to the preparation of the dancer. Success comes from preparation. It comes through practice, and perhaps, most importantly, it comes from the ritual that sets up the dance moves. A ballerina can complete a pirouette only if she enters the move with the correct footwork. The correct footwork comes from ritualistic practice.

Painters can only apply the colors and shadings as prescribed if they hold the brush correctly and experiment with a variety of different color mixtures and palettes. The sculptor must develop a delicate touch with the chisel. These skills come from practice.

Good teachers teach through rituals. Warm-up exercises in dance and sports are such rituals. In golf and basketball, players must develop a pre-shot routine that they repeat. It is the set-up that creates the posture for success. A good set-up comes from practicing the set-up as a ritual.

Practicing rituals teach us about ourselves. Some days we have more talent as therapists than others. Some days artists find their zones, and other days they don't seem to be as talented. Tiger Woods, the champion golfer, often comments, "I didn't bring my A game with me today" to explain this phenomenon of some days being "on" and of others being "off."

When we practice a ritual, we can learn about where we are in relation to our talent and our best selves. Rituals can help us become aware of our feelings and our strengths. If we feel we have lost our talent, a ritual will help us find it. And if not, a ritual will help us know what to expect from ourselves on this day.

Art, Emotion, Reason, and Ritual

Carol Cole is a frequently exhibited artist. Her primary image is the breast. Her art has a southern, yet universal theme. Her art highlights the fascination with and power of the breast, juxtaposed with how easily its nurturing function is ignored, punished, and taken for granted. Cole spent much of her thirties in a mental hospital, suffering from some version of psychosis. At that time her art was tight, obsessive, detailed, and difficult to interpret.

According to Cole, she found sanity through her art when one day she illustrated her fears. They were symbolic conceptual images that she could see detached from herself. Once she saw them apart from herself, she understood that her fears belonged to everyone. With this new perspective on her fears, she could develop skills to cope with them. The more she expressed them in drawings, the further she separated herself from her fears, the more mentally strong she became. When she considered the fears to be the sum of who she was and uniquely hers, she felt crazy. When she saw them as various forms of the breast, she saw her fears were universal. She first saw these fears in women; subsequently she saw them in men and children as well.

Winnicott (1989) writes about this process as developing the inner "good-enough mother." Others call it the development of the observing ego. This is the ability to separate and reflect on one's self, to see one's self, and to judge, nurture, and control the self. The development of an internal "good-enough mother" requires this detaching from one's feelings and behavior that Cole describes in her artwork. Artists take on this detached perspective that allows them to observe and express their feelings when they work and reflect on them as expressed in their creation.

Rutledge in his book, *Embracing Fear* (2002), and in his coauthored book, *Life Without Ed* (2003), discusses a four-step model to emotional well-being. The first step is to understand that what might appear as crazy behavior does make emotional sense. All feelings and behavior have a context. Knowing the context helps us understand ourselves. The second step is to separate or "dis-identify" with one's behavior and feelings. This "dis-identification" process helps us see that the behavior does not define or encompass the self. This is the step that often requires art and imagination. For people suffering with eating disorders, he suggests that they name the disorder. "Ed" is an example of a name that is often used for this purpose. Then, he encourages people to have conversations with Ed, to write these down, to draw Ed or sing songs about Ed, and so forth. Steps three and four are setting positive goals and learning to succeed, respectively. The critical step to recovery, however, is the second step in which art and imagination are used to develop detachment from the behavior and feelings. This detachment, this observing ego, or "good-enough mother," creates the perspective necessary to understand the emotional reasons for the behavior and to develop new behaviors and new emotional paths to take the place of the old ones.

In chapter 2, we discovered that emotions have more connections to each other and the body than to the cognition of the neocortex. Art promotes the connection between cognition and emotion. This is the same function that rituals perform. Rituals can create new emotional pathways that promote emotional health and expand the connection between thinking and feeling, so that thought can serve feeling, so that feelings can make sense, so that feelings can be seen as universal, so that thoughts can help feelings find a constructive expression.

Research and Emotional Rituals in Psychotherapy

In chapter 5, we will discuss Steven Stosny's compassion program and his HEALS technique. His research on his program demonstrates the effectiveness of a ritual.

Stosny maintained that much of the content of his 12-session program was filler and basically irrelevant. The primary intervention tool was the HEALS technique. Its purpose is to take an individual from anger through sadness to compassion for the self and others. In every session, the material served as an excuse to support and continue the ritual's daily practice.

Research on the Duluth-model batterers programs has demonstrated that individuals treated in the Duluth-model programs are as likely or more likely to batter than they were prior to treatment (Harrell, 1991). Stosny (1995) conducted research in his area, comparing his treatment programs to the Duluth-model programs.

After the first session of the Duluth-model programs, 50% of the participants did not return. Only 10% completed the program. This is compared to a 75% completion rate of Stosny's compassion program. Of the 10%, 90% re-offended within 1 year. Of the 75% that completed Stosny's compassion program, 90% did not re-offend within 1 year.

If Stosny is correct, that the HEALS technique is his primary treatment, then this ritual was effective.

Other research has been done on rituals like the CALMS technique (see chapter 6). In *The Relaxation Response* (Benson, 1975), the author documents the effectiveness of this practice.

The Brain is Plastic

It has long been taken for granted that a child's brain is adaptable and when injured can compensate for severe brain trauma. It is not uncommon for brain surgeons to remove half of a child's brain in what's called a hemispherectomy and to find that same child talking, running, jumping, and doing well in school after the surgery. The child's brain is miraculously resilient, adaptable, and malleable. This is not so for the adult brain.

If we as adults had a hemispherectomy, we would not recover well at all. It has long been assumed that once we reach the age of 25 or 26 our brains are no longer changeable. Neuroplasticity was thought to be reserved for the young.

In the early 1990s (the decade President G. H. Bush designated as the decade of the brain), researchers began probing the limits of neuroplasticity, first in animals (Merzenich, 2000) and snails (Kandel, 1995) and subsequently with monkeys (Taub, Uswatte, & Pidikiti, 1999).

Only in the late 1990s, did scientists begin to produce evidence that the human adult brain was malleable. Several researchers have now demonstrated that experience, especially ritualistic behavior repetition, changes the brain.

One study of note was conducted by Eleanor McGuire (2000) of University College of London. She studied the brains of London cabbies. To earn a license to drive a cab, London taxi drivers must pass a stringent test that appraises their knowledge of the shortest route from place to place in London. Preparation for the exam usually takes two years. Cabbies call it "being on the knowledge."

McGuire believed that such extensive knowledge would be reflected by the size of the part of the hippocampus that stores directional memory. She collected magnetic resonant images of 16 London male cabbies, ages 32 to 62, and compared them to images of 50 ordinary right-handed men in the same age range. She found what she was looking for. The brains were the same except for the hippocampus, the part of the brain in charge of memory. The back segment of the hippocampus (which is the part of the brain that houses directional memory) was significantly larger in the cabdrivers. In fact, the longer a man had been a cabdriver, the larger the rear segment of the hippocampus was and the smaller the front part of the hippocampus. Several scientists have confirmed such brain changes in adults (Schwartz, 2004).

One such study is particularly relevant to our question about rituals. That question is: Can rituals help? We can see that emotions can change brain chemicals, but, even more to the point, can rituals change the brain? Jeffrey Schwartz (2004) devised a ritual treatment for obsessive-compulsive disordered (OCD) patients. His was a four-step ritual that was primarily cognitive behavioral. His ritual did not focus on emotions as do those in this book. For his mnemonic, he used four words that began with "Re:" (1) Relabel, (2) Reattribute, (3) Refocus, (4) Revalue. His goal in this treatment was to make use of the Buddhist construct of mindfulness. It was his contention that these steps were essentially the aspects of that construct.

Relabeling, the first step, means identify the obsessive urge or thought as the product of a brain malfunction. Once seen in this way, it is easier to separate one's self from the brain and what it is doing. Relabeling enables OCD clients to understand that this urge comes from their OCD, not from them. They are able to begin detaching from their obsessive worries and urges with this first step.

The second step, Reattribute, is taking away the self as the cause of the obsessions and reattributing the cause to malfunctioning in the brain. These obviously aberrant messages come from a brain disease. The brain is going to function this way. This is not the fault of OCD clients. Just because the brain pushes these thoughts into the participants' head doesn't mean they have to accept them. They can fight back.

The third step in the Schwartz OCD ritual is Refocus. This is the pivotal step in the four-step process. Schwartz (2004) called it "the core step" for the whole therapy. The job here is to refocus attention on adaptive behavior. This is not an attempt to banish a thought. It is instead the step that initiates a new thought about pleasant, healthy behavior. In this step, a good circuit is substituted for a bad circuit. Here, willpower is required. "This is the step, more than any other, that produces changes in the brain" (p. 86).

The final step, Revaluing, circles back to the first. This is a deeper form of Relabeling. "It was intended to enhance patient's use of mindfulness. It is wise as opposed to unwise attention. . . . In the case of OCD, wise attention means quickly recognizing the disturbing thoughts as senseless, as false, as errant brain signals not even worth the gray matter they rode in on" (p. 88).

By the late 1990s, using this ritual, Schwartz and his colleagues achieved an astounding 80% success rate, with no relapse in OCD clients. In developing his four-step ritual, Schwartz studied the brains of eighteen OCD drug-free patients. At that time, he was primarily using step three, Refocus, as his treatment. Of the 18 patients, 12 significantly improved with 10-week group treatment. The PET scans of these 12 patients showed significant changes from pre- to posttreatment. The right and left caudate nucleus was much less active in the post-treatments scans. In the before-treatment scans, there was a high level of correlated activity among the three parts of the OCD brain triad: the caudate nucleus, the orbital frontal cortex, and the thalamus in the right hemisphere. In the post-treatment scans, this coordinated brain activity was not present. The OCD brain lock had been broken.

John Teasdale and colleagues used a similar treatment process for depression, teaching mindfulness to depressed clients. He called his treatment "mindful experiencing/being." His treatment was to help clients understand that "thoughts are not facts" and "I am not my thoughts." His next step was similar to the Schwartz third step, Refocus. In this step, Teasdale asked his clients to attend to healthier associations.

When Teasdale studied the mindfulness treatment of depression, he focused on rates of relapse. He enrolled 145 patients, ages 18 to 65. All patients had experienced at least two episodes of depression within the last 5 years; none was taking medications for depression. The treatment consisted of 2-hour weekly group sessions, with homework between sessions for 8 weeks. He randomly assigned half of the participants to his mindful experiencing/being treatment and half to standard cognitive-behavioral treatment. In the treatment group, there was a 44% reduction in the rate of relapse as compared to the control cognitive-behavior group.

Perhaps even more impressive than these results is the use of similar ritualized treatment with patients suffering from Tourette's syndrome. This is an illness that is similar to OCD. The patient suffers from irrepressible urges to move or speak in bizarre ways. Speech outbursts are often out-of-character cursing or name-calling. Outbursts of movements might be simple tics, wild arm swings, or episodes of constant eye blinking. John Piacentini had notions similar to Schwartz's, that Tourette's had much in common with OCD and that the same brain circuitry was involved.

He designed a treatment that he called "awareness training," which shared similar elements with the Schwartz "mindfulness training." Again, the key element to treatment was akin to the third step, the Refocus step, in the

Schwartz version. Piacentini combined awareness training with what he called "habit modulation." When Tourette's clients feel the urge to move or speak, the program's tenets instructed them to substitute a safe intentional movement that was slower and less intense for, let's say, a tic.

Seventeen children suffering from Tourette's were part of Piacentini and Chang's (2001) study. Those who received awareness training alone had a 10% improvement in tic severity. Those who received the two-pronged training, awareness plus habit modulation training, experienced a 30% reduction in tic severity and 56% improvement in tic related impairment.

The main elements that the Schwartz "mindfulness training," the Teasdale "mindful experiencing/being," and the Piacentini "awareness and habit modulation training" have in common are: (1) identifying the pathological process as a brain malfunction; (2) refocusing the brain in a different healthy direction; and (3) initiating healthy thoughts and behaviors.

All the rituals I propose here have these elements in common with Schwartz, Teasdale, and Piacentini. What they offer that is different is a particular refocus on a particular emotion that seems most likely to be effective in breaking what Schwartz calls "a brain lock" and what I call "an emotional knot." We'll discuss this later.

The three preceding studies demonstrate the power of rituals. Drug therapy has already demonstrated that feelings are tied to neuromodulators and that changing neuromodulators via drugs changes feelings. The corollary, then, is obvious. Changing feelings also changes brain chemicals.

These studies, however, demonstrate that one can change the brain's structure by practicing rituals. In the case of the London cabbies, the anterior hippocampus is enlarged. In the case of OCD, PET scans of the patients demonstrated that the wiring of the OCD brain triangle can be broken. Although Teasdale and Piacentini did not have PET scans, their findings support Schwartz's and McGuire's. Our brains are plastic, and with repeated rituals, we can choose to change our brains as well as their chemicals.

But the Light Bulb Must Want to Change

The old joke is: "How many therapists does it take to change a light bulb?" The answer is: "One, but the light bulb has to really want to change." There is no therapy that will be successful with all people. That patient variable is a constant. We cannot escape the fact that a successful patient must be motivated. And a motivated patient often recovers despite, or with the help of, therapy.

The following research demonstrates the effort that it takes to change the brain. The first set of studies concerning effort is about constraint-induced movement therapy for chronic stroke victims. Years of sometimes cruel research on animals, especially monkeys, had demonstrated that, in a brain-injured mammal that has lost the use of, say, the right arm, that restraining the left arm, the "good" arm, so that it cannot be used, forces the animal to use what appears to be a useless right arm. In time, the brain develops new neural routes, and the mammal, through great effort and repeated practice, gains use of the once useless arm.

As early as 1967, Larry Anderson tried constraint-induced movement therapy (Schwartz, 2004) with human chronic stroke victims with more than one year of limb paralysis, first with four patients, then again with twenty-four. These participants all believed that they would never be able to use their paralyzed arm. There was substantial improvement in all the patients. The scientific community and the clinical community dismissed these ideas out-of-hand for the following reasons. First, it was the official position of the American Stroke Association that rehab for chronic stroke victims should primarily include work with the parts of the body that have motor function. Second, it was the consensus of the scientific community at that time that the adult brain could not generate new neural patterns in adults. These two reasons combined with the third. And that was that most of the results about neuroplasticity in animal brains came from Edward Taub. Taub was convicted of animal cruelty because of his treatment of the now-famous Silver Spring monkeys in a controversial trial. Rehab specialists were reluctant to put into practice ideas that came from his work.

Whether Taub mistreated the monkeys in his care is a matter for another forum, but the implications of Taub's experiments on the brains of monkeys, documenting their ability to regenerate neural paths that facilitate movement, were ignored for years.

It was not until the late 1990s that constraint-induced movement was used widely to treat patients with strokes. The results have been uniformly positive. As late as 1990, it was assumed that after 1 year the brain could not recover lost function. Rehabilitation, therefore, ended after 1 year. After that, further rehabilitation was assumed unproductive. Because Taub continued to espouse the notion of brain neuroplasticity and constraint-induced movement therapy, we know the brain can be rewired with a great deal of practice and effort.

The treatment is usually done involving participants with one paralyzed arm. The useful arm is constrained in a sling. This forces participants to use the useless arms as best they can. Imagine the frustration they must tolerate. Imagine the force of will these participants must generate. Imagine the emotion put behind the neural firings in the brain to stimulate the use of the paralyzed arm. And participants endure this for 90% of their waking hours for 14 days, without relief. On each of the 10 weekdays of this 14-day period, they receive 6 hours of therapy, pushing about objects with what had been a useless arm. They eat meals without the use of their good arm; they throw balls; play board and card games, using their "bad" arm. In a game of checkers, participants may labor to pick up a checker for 30 minutes. Therapists offer encouragement and tailor the next task so that it is challenging, but doable. This takes great effort and patience from participants, therapists, and onlookers.

The next research program demonstrating the effort required to change the brain involves children with specific language impairment (SLI).

Treatment of patients (usually children) with SLI also has demonstrated that the brain can be remodeled. The theory base of current treatment is that (perhaps because of ear infections in early childhood) the sound distinction part of the brain (the auditory cortex) did not develop properly. Consequently, it takes SLI patients a long time for their brains to process a phoneme (a sound shift). This is the period of time (one-third to one-fifth of a second) that it usually takes for us to process the length of a whole syllable, not just a sound of a short phoneme, like "ba."

Treatment involves asking these patients to listen to tapes of stretched-out speech. In this speech, the sounds and phonemes are said slowly. After a month of this treatment, children's speech comprehension advanced two years. The training consisted of 3 hours a day practice, every weekday, plus everyday play at home, with computer games using modified slow speech. This again requires great effort and practice, but it is not surprising that this is effective with children, because children's brains have always been considered malleable or plastic.

The third set of studies centers primarily on the adult brain that until 1990 was considered not plastic or malleable. The patients in these studies are participants suffering from focal-hand dystonia. This is a neurological disorder that affects people who have highly skilled hands that can make rapid repetitive finger movements. Often those suffering from focal-hand dystonia are musicians, or keyboard users.

The theory behind the treatment for focal-hand dystonia is that nearly simultaneous coincident-repetitive inputs from the brain to the fingers might cause the primary sensory cortex to lose its ability to identify which finger is being stimulated. The part of the brain that moves the ring finger may also stimulate the middle finger to move (Byl, et al., 1996). Previous experiments on animals suggested that it takes 10,000 to 100,000 repetitions to degrade a memory in animals. The task for patients of focal-hand dystonia would be to first degrade the pathologically overlapping impulses that confuse various fingers when the brain stimulates movement, and then to rebuild a new circuit with the correct associations. The treatment task would be to have the correct finger move slowly and deliberately, separate from the other fingers. This requires hour after hour of sitting and slowly practicing. The old neural network is degraded, and a new one is built. Byl (1996) and Candia (1999) did just that with accomplished musicians who were suffering from focal-hand dystonia. All of them improved. Most returned to professional performance after treatment. Therapy was successful in improving hand coordination in all patients.

There's another catch. And that is, if you stop practicing, the brain returns to its original state. In Germany, Bogdan Draganski taught twelve people how to juggle. Draganski photographed the brain at the end of 3 months of practice. The pictures showed that the grey matter in the mid-temporal (hMT/v5) area and in the left posterior intraparietal sulcus had significantly expanded. At this point, the same participants stopped juggling and ceased practice. Three months later, Draganski photographed the participants' brains. The last set of pictures found that their brains had returned to their previous size, and the subjects had lost most of their talent for juggling.

The point of all these studies is that building new brain networks that change emotional habits requires incredible effort, determination, and practice. Dedicated patients that practice a ritual likely will build new neural pathways and change their brain chemistry. The light bulb has to want to change. We must practice a great deal to learn a new emotional skill, and we must keep practicing to maintain that skill.

The problem with this line of thinking is that it can lead us to blaming the victim. Of course, will, by itself, cannot produce new brain circuits or new brain chemistry. There are passive mental events and intentional ones. Sometimes the passive mental acts or mental structures cannot be overcome by intention. But that does not mean that our will or choice or the intentional focus of our attention has no power. It's not an all-or-nothing matter. Will won't stop the voices or the hallucinations in schizophrenia, but John Nash, the schizophrenic subject of A Beautiful Mind, proved that one can will oneself to ignore the voices.

Depression is a disease of the will. For a depressed person, willing, choosing, and wanting is dangerous. It involves the hope of success, and the depressed person feels he or she cannot afford that hope. When depression is mixed in with other psychological problems, like OCD or agoraphobia, the will to get better is diminished. Well-being comes not just from chemicals or neurons. It comes from the support of friends and family. It comes from competent professional caring and medical support. It can come from fate turning our fortunes in love or money.

Even if we assume Schwartz is correct, that his four-step ritual cures 80% of his patients with no relapse, what about the remaining 20%? Though we cannot be sure what they needed that they did not get from Schwartz and his colleagues, it is possible that they needed more time and attention for the process of recovery to unfold. If, for example, their OCD was contaminated with grief from the loss of a parent, before they could develop the desire and determination to get better, they first would have to get through the grieving process. There is no ritual that can take the place of time and a healthy therapeutic alliance. Effective listening or "being present for" always is the most important tool of a good therapist's toolbox.

Just as successful therapy requires a committed client, we also need to be patient until our clients can find the courage to hope and want that will lead to the discovery of their determination to get well.

The Problem is the Solution

The problem, which is the subject here, is the fact that we easily get stuck in one emotion. The reason for this is the well-known neurological premise, "What's fired together is wired together." An example of this is a twenty-something-year-old male client named Gary. His girlfriend recently dumped him. "She was the one," he said. "I thought this was it. I can't believe she did this. I am hurt by this, but that's not all that's here. When this happened I began to grieve all over again about all of my losses: my father's death when I was 18; my torn muscle at 16, which stopped my football career; my first girlfriend's suicide. Well, she wasn't my dating girlfriend. She was more a friend, but I loved her. If my mind is not thinking about one of these things, it is thinking about one of the others. I'm stuck here, and I can't seem to get out of this place."

Gary's depression occurred because his sad losses are associated with each another. They are wired together in his brain. When he thinks of one, all the others come tumbling out with it. When he experiences a new loss, it becomes attached to the old ones. And Gary gets even more stuck.

It is the same with music. This is the reason we can play name that tune. Someone plays a bar or two of a song, and our mind plays the rest of it for us. What's wired together, fires together.

This neurological phenomenon that gets us stuck in sadness, like Gary, or helps us name that tune is also the same thing that can rescue us from our emotional stuck place. All we have to do is refocus and attend to a memory with a different and new emotional riff. When we shift our attention in this way, the principle of what's wired together is fired together takes us in a new emotional direction. This then becomes our solution.

The difficulty with this is that, too often, we cannot find a posture or a platform where we can shift our focus. For example, Gary was addicted to being in the center of a drama. He loved the action. He hated being placed at the margins. But as the key man, the essential, but-for person, neither we nor Gary can find the space and perspective to move our minds to a new subject.

This is where the artist has the advantage. Artists thrive at the margins. From the margins, they can easily shift their foci. If they can't paint this picture, they can turn, find a new perspective, and paint that one, whereas people who are at the center of a crisis cannot shift their attention.

Gary is an example of this. Gary said, "I'm bored with this new job. It's 8 to 5. I'm ahead of my bosses. There are no crises to manage, no fires to put out. I'm just biding my time until something comes along that absorbs my attention. I don't want to go home to my empty house. I liked it better when my job filled my life."

Now that Gary is on the margins and not in the center, he doesn't know what to do with himself. His interests are work and mating. He wants both of them to absorb him. He has no idea how to be an artist, to stand at the margins and create, choosing among his various interests. He does not know where he can profitably shift his focus. He seems lost if he is not in the center of things.

When life casts us to its margins, we have the opportunity to use this place to practice our rituals and to develop a new emotional repertoire. The margins are our briar patch, and a new ritual can be our discovered treasure.

Designing a Ritual

Clearly rituals work because practice of a new skill can rewire the brain. This requires an effective ritual, a determined client and lots of practice. Consider the Schwartz four-step ritual. The thing it leaves out is any connection to the emotions. Steps 1, 2, and 4 in Schwartz's ritual are basically the same. He called Step 1, Relabeling; Step 2, Reattribute; and Step 4, Revaluing. These three steps simply remind the client that the OCD is not them; it is a malfunctioning brain. While I agree that the client needs to separate their identity from their symptoms and that it would help to give clients some education about how OCD works in the brain, I don't think it needs to be a part of a ritual. These steps, by themselves, do not change brain chemicals or shape the brain structure. The real crux of his ritual is his step three, Refocus. This is exactly what all the emotion rituals in this book do. They refocus the brain. In our emotion rituals, we refocus on a new emotion to break the brain lock of the former emotion or set of emotions. The problem with Schwartz's refocus is that he doesn't offer direction on where to refocus, except to say "a pleasant, familiar, good habit."

Let's consider how we might use our emotion principle to build a better OCD ritual. Of course, it will have to include refocusing. Schwartz demonstrated that piece was essential. Yes, I think treatment should include some information about the malfunctioning brain triad of the caudate nucleus, the orbital frontal lobe, and the anterior cingulate gyrus and how these get wrapped up in one another, locking the brain into compulsive urges. But I don't think this must be part of a ritual. OCD patients know their brains aren't working right. Each OCD episode reminds them of that.

And of course, we should refocus toward an emotion that is not fear, since fear is the major emotional foundation for OCD. Consider R I G H T as an acronym for our five steps. R, then, would be, "Refocus on something you want." This begins the ritual with the emotion of desire. The letter I might direct us toward joy and the sense of well-being. I might represent, "Insist that you remember you are not your fears. You are a valuable lovable person." Next, we need an antidote to fear. Our third step, symbolized by G, might be, "Go slow. Relax." This engages the relaxation response. The fourth step might push us into the emotion of surprise/wonder. The letter H might be, "Hold on to wonder." Then T, the last step, might be an action step moving the person into a behavior. "Take-off" might work as the last step.

The whole ritual would then be something like this:

 Step 1: R would be Refocus. Shift your attention to something you want and desire. Break the brain lock of worry and fear with your passion.

 Step 2: Insist that you remember you are not your fears. You are a valuable lovable person. Recall a time when you succeeded and you felt good about yourself. Perhaps it is a graduation, a dance recital, or a winning game. Feel proud of yourself. This provides an antidote to shame and the beginning of self-awareness.

 Step 3: Go slow. Relax. Release the tension from your body. Begin with your feet and move up. Take a deep breath, breathe naturally and easily. Focus your mind on the memory of your success and your value. Center yourself in that value. This engages the relaxation response and turns off fear.

 Step 4: Hold on to wonder. Be curious. Let control slip away. Watch how fate works. Prepare to act without controlling the response. Let events unfold. Discover in these events things you wanted that you did not expect to get.

 Step 5: Take-off. Go get what you want. Make a plan and take action. Focus on desiring and achieving your desire. This step engages us in behavior instead of thought, fear, and worry. Act.

While that may work well for OCD patients, consider eating-disorder patients and sex addicts. This is what they do. They feel fear and refocus on something that they want. Sexual excitement turns on the parasympathetic part of the autonomic nervous system. You cannot be turned on and afraid.

Hunger for food does the same thing. You cannot desire food and be afraid at the same time. Eating-disorder patients have the same OCD brain lock. Their brains simply shift from fear to want and they get stuck in their food appetite. I would guess that the same three brain parts (the caudate nucleus, the orbital frontal lobe in the anterior cingulate) are the culprits in an eating disorder as well. The ritual we designed for OCD is, in fact, exactly what individuals with eating disorders do. The refocus step is where they begin. They feel fear, and they refocus on something they want: food. In the bulimic, the focus is on eating food. For the anorectic, the focus is on not eating, thus starving, therefore keeping food as the primary subject of the brain, canceling out fear or shame with hunger. The anorectic uses starving just as we use the second step, the I step, "Insist on your worth." The anorectic is proud of the self-discipline that starving requires. Her thinness is testimony to her worth.

If we use the R I G H T ritual with eating-disorder clients, we would be prescribing what they already do all too well. Let's imagine we were designing a ritual for eating-disorder clients, using the principles we learned from Schwartz. Consider S H I F T for our acronym.

The first step might be:

 Step 1: Stop. Disobey the eating-disorder voice. Separate yourself from your eating disorder. Remember the eating-disorder urge is a brain lock. It is not you. Resist the urge. This engages anger.

 Step 2: Hang out. Relax. Let go of mastery or perfection. Just be yourself, your messed-up self that feels and cannot control life or the world. Be yourself. Control only your breath. Breathe deeply, slowly, and naturally. Let peace come.

 Step 3: Include fate. Instead of over-controlling yourself, open up to fate. Be curious about how things will work out if you just focus on your health—your real health—and listen to what your body feels. When it is hungry, eat. When it is full, stop. Let your mind and heart feel. Emotions won't drown you. The good thing about feelings is that they are always changing. Be curious. Watch how your feelings evolve. Watch fate work.

 Step 4: Find some things you want that are healthy. Not one thing, but things. Plural. Consider which one of these healthy actions you want to pursue now, an action that will give you balance and bring inner harmony.

 Step 5: Take off. Go after the healthy habit you have chosen.

You can design rituals for particular emotional problems and for particular patients. In following chapters, we will discuss which feelings are healthy resolutions and which might not be. This information is essential to the building of an effective ritual.

Some of the rituals presented in this book, like the CALMS ritual (chapter 6) and the HEART ritual (chapter 5), have a great deal of support and will seem familiar to the reader. Others will seem more foreign and will take some time and perhaps some personal practice in order to appreciate their effectiveness. Perhaps once readers understand the various healthy emotional patterns, they may wish to develop their own rituals, as I have, or improve on the ones presented here.

Compassion, Gratitude, Praise, and Peace

We should not forget or dismiss emotions that make up most religious rituals. They have worked for centuries and still do. Most religious rituals include one or a combination of these emotions: compassion, gratitude, praise, or peace. Peace is a combination of anger management and engaging the trance, as in the CALMS ritual. Compassion is an attachment that takes one out of one's own emotions and connects one to the feelings of others. Gratitude is a combination of humility and joy. It is the celebration of a gift (joy) and the recognition that perhaps it was undeserved (shame). Gratitude also shifts one from an internal focus to an external one. Praise is similar to gratitude. It is joy in the strength, competence, and success of another, thus a shift of focus away from the self and personal feelings. On NBC's *Today Show* on September 2, 2003, reporter Ann Curry remarked to Rabbi Harold Kushner that one could not feel sad and blessed at the same time. This confirms the basic theory of this book.

The problem with these traditional mind cleaners is that they can be used as a denial or a repression defense. Greenberg (2002) is fond of saying you cannot leave a place before you have arrived. Before one uses any of these religious rituals to move on to a positive mood, it is important to feel, express, and acknowledge one's other emotions. If we experience our dark emotions first, the religious rituals that engage compassion, gratitude, praise, and peace are healthy, useful emotional tools.

Summary and Conclusion

The point is that rituals are a useful resource to the psychotherapy process. This book does not suggest a new psychotherapy. Rather, it organizes information, which many research psychologists have known for a long time, into rituals that become tools for the psychotherapy alliance. These tools empower clients. They center the process of change around the client's work outside the therapy hour and inside the client's daily life.

These rituals offer clients a chance to practice by themselves what they are learning about in therapy, outside therapy. Rituals give clients a process that provides them an opportunity to practice and grow from their personal work. Rituals help clients disengage from the productive process of routine work and move toward the artistic process of reflection, self-awareness, and self-expression. Rituals give clients a tool that they can use, independent of the therapist, to check their own emotional strength or temperature. Rituals create a platform that helps clients prepare themselves for emotional work in relationships.

Emotional rituals can help us master the art of self-awareness and emotional self-expression. These can help us make healthy links among emotions and avoid pathological emotional traps. They can help us develop healthy emotional patterns and emotional self-control, without numbing all-important feelings.

Becoming masters of ourselves and our emotions is the point of psychotherapy. That requires practice, and emotional rituals create a structure for that practice.

CHAPTER 4

How the Mind Feels
The Basic Emotions

Effective psychotherapists change a client's brain chemistry all the time, though they might not know it. Thoughts, feelings, ideas, memories, and images in our minds all have neurological locations and correlating neurochemicals. When we therapists mess with these, we are affecting the inside of a human brain.

Psychotherapists need to know what their interventions are doing to their clients' brains. To do that, they must know about the neurostructure of the brain and the neurohormones that make up the brain's chemistry. This is the reason for this chapter and the reason for the review of each emotion's specific neurobiology in the chapters that follow.

This field is quickly changing. Although this book describes neurostructures and neurochemicals as if they were separate entities, they are not. These distinctions may help explain how the brain works, using linear ways of understanding, but that is not how the brain actually works.

Therapists generally do not prescribe medications. Therefore, knowing whether the body is responding to a short-lived, fast-acting neurotransmitter or a longer-lasting blood stream delivered neurohormone is irrelevant. Even texts that teach brain chemistry blur the distinction between these two (Olson, 2001).[4] For our purposes, we will call all these chemicals neuromodulators. Another qualification is that any rendition of the known workings of the brain is out-of-date once it is written. New neuromodulators are discovered and previously unknown neurological relationships understood every day. The technological advances of the various radiological-imaging techniques have made this one of science's and medicine's most exciting fields. I apologize in advance, therefore, for my sometimes simplistic description of the workings of the human brain and how it experiences feelings.

This chapter reviews the functions of the neuromodulators known, at this writing, to be active in the expression of emotion. The chapter begins by listing and discussing the primary neuromodulators. I present these, first, with a story demonstrating what happens when the neurostructure is at work, followed by a brief discussion of the structure and function of the neurocircuitry.

The Emotional Neuromodulators

Catecholamines

Fourteen-year-old Bobby was a golfer who regularly shot par. He aspired to play tournament golf and hoped someday to play on the P.G.A. tour. He consulted me because I'm a golfer and a psychologist, and I played competitive sports as a youth. Here is what he told me:

> I don't know what goes on with me. I don't play well when I play with my little brother. I'm bored, I guess. I seem to need competition to be at my best. When I play with my friends or my dad, I play great. But at a tournament when they announce my name as next to tee off, something happens to me. My nerves—I can barely focus. I feel faint. I always seem to blow that first shot. I do terrible for some time—bogies, double bogies for maybe the first six holes. By the ninth hole, I'm out of contention. I can't possibly win. Then, I calm down. I can shoot three or four under par on the back nine. But that's too little, too late. I don't understand what happens to me.

Though I didn't explain it this way to Bobby, the answer is catecholamines. (With Bobby, I discussed the "inverted U" effect of stress that Yerkes-Dodson (1908) described, which explained his behavior.) An increase in dopamine (DA) and norepinephrine (NE) catecholamines increase performance at low levels. But as these chemicals accumulate with increased pressure above a certain threshold in the brain, performance suffers (Buck, 1999).

High levels of two of the catecholamines, norepinephrine and dopamine, increase anxiety, and high levels of NE catecholamines alone are associated with depression.

Dopamine (DA)

Bobby's tournament play improved. In a recent event, Bobby had the lead by two strokes when he finished his last holes. He was excited about the prospect that he might win. Then, as others finished, Bobby got the news that he came in fourth. He was disappointed.

Internally, Bobby's dopamine level fluctuated with his excitement. Dopamine is the body's pleasure accountant. It has to do with expectations. When our expectations are exceeded (as when Bobby had the lead for the first time in tournament play), our dopamine levels are high. Extra dopamine comes with good news. When expectations are not met (as when Bobby found out he didn't win), dopamine levels go down. This sends us out to search for a new reward. (The lowered levels of dopamine sent Bobby to the practice tee.) Dopamine is associated with curiosity (Panksepp, 1998). Low levels of dopamine are associated with addiction.

Monoamine Oxidase (MAO)

Alice was consulting me about her 8-year-old son, Todd.

"He had a good year in school," she said. "But things changed last month after he attended a party for his soccer team. He played goalie, and in the last game of the season, he didn't block the opposing team's winning goal. Prior to the party, Todd was outgoing and friendly. But suddenly, at this party, he isolated himself. He has been painfully shy ever since. What happened?"

Although I didn't share this explanation with Alice, what happened was that Todd's brain was overwhelmed with monoamine oxidase. MAO breaks down the other amines–the DA and NE catecholamines, as well as serotonin (5-HT). Presence of these other amines creates euphoric effects. When high levels of MAO are present, low levels of the other amines are as well. Hence, drugs that inhibit MAO production can be used as antidepressants. High levels of MAO are related to introversion and social isolation (Buck, 1999). When MAO levels are high, the sympathetic system is usually dominant. The body is being aroused by one or more of the following: fear, anger, surprise, or desire.

Endorphins

I love my dog, Greco, and if the number of times he licks my face is any indication, Greco loves me. Like many therapists, I have lower-back pain. Either I hurt in the morning while I stretch my body, or I neglect to stretch my body and consequently hurt all day. One of my daily exercises is to lie on three towels rolled into a single roll placed in the small of my back, and for five minutes, I lie there in pain. I had been doing this for 2 years before adding Greco to our family. Now, as I lie on the towels in pain, I invite Greco to lie beside me with his head on my shoulder. Greco always obliges. Somehow, with Greco by my side, my back doesn't hurt as much. How could that be—possibly because behavior related to attachment and bonding releases endorphins (along with oxytocin and vasopressin).

Endorphins are endogenous body chemicals that act like morphine. They are the brain's own opiates. In fact, Beta endorphin is arguably the most powerful pain-killing substance available. It is more addictive than heroin and one hundred times more powerful than morphine (Panksepp, 1993). Endorphins are associated with tender, loving, physical contact.

Endorphins are a part of the peptide neurochemical system. A combination of amino acids creates an endorphin. An endorphin is a string of these 16 amino acids made up of 91 parts. The first 41 of these are adrenocorticotropic hormones (ACTH). The next 50 are amino acids, numbers 42 to 60, and constitute the melanocyte-stimulating hormone (MSH). (Incidentally, MSH darkens the skin when exposed to ultraviolet light.) And numbers 61 to 91 constitute the powerful pain reliever, beta-endorphin.

Panksepp (1993) speculated that we can be addicted to love. He also believed that drug addicts use drugs, because they do not have the skills or the social resources to create endorphin flow in their bodies. Consequently, this addiction further impairs their social skills needed to create attachments. Once they begin to use external painkillers, addicts do not need human attachments. They become antisocial and lose their sense of shame.

Greco is my opiate in the morning.

Serotonin (5-HT)

Remember Bobby, the 14-year-old golfer? I told Bobby the secret of the golfer's psychological universe. When he consulted me after his next tournament, this is what he said:

> I'm not exactly sure what happened, but when I got up on the first tee, I did what you told me. (Exactly what I told Bobby will remain a secret.) Suddenly, I knew I could do it. I was relaxed. I was confident. I knew what I was going to do. My focus was clear. My first drive followed the fairway irrigation pipeline, right down the middle. I played well—not good enough to win—I placed third. I'm not sure what happened on that first tee. Can you tell me so that I can count on doing it again?

My response to Bobby related to visualization. But what really happened was that Bobby flooded his brain with serotonin. Serotonin is also called 5-hydroxytriptaimine (5- HT). It is particularly associated with ego-strength and confidence. It helps us cope with rejection (Kramer, 1993). It helps the body relax as it activates the parasympathetic system, thus promoting relaxation and sleep (Buck, 1988). It affects social leadership, impulse control, and dominance with low levels of aggression. Low levels of serotonin are related to a high sensitivity to insult and rejection (or short fuses). We can positively correlate serotonin levels with social acceptance and respect and also connect it, in a negative sense, to shame and social failure (Panksepp, 1993).

Cholecystokinin (CCK)

Ralph had a weight problem. He consulted me to determine if there was a psychological reason for his inability to control his eating. This is what he said about his disordered eating:

> I do fine for a couple of days, and then something goes wrong at work. I get nervous, and I hit the all-you-can-eat buffets. Or, I go to a party with people I don't know. I get anxious, and I stand around the food table and eat. Whenever I get afraid or anxious, I use food to comfort me, and I don't know why.

The answer to Ralph's disordered eating has something to do with cholecystokinin. CCK is a peptide that regulates the appetite (Loumaye, Thorner, & Cutt, 1982). And CCK is also strongly associated with fear (Bradwejm, 1993). This peptide increases blood flow to the limbic system, where the fight/flight regulator, the amygdala, is located. When humans are injected with CCK, they report strong feelings of anxiety and fear (Reiman, Fusselman, Fox, & Raichle, 1989).

Ralph probably has a high dose of CCK whenever he is afraid, thus stimulating his appetite. He eats food, hoping to satisfy some part of his brain and perhaps comfort his fears.

Oxytocin (OXY)

I had been seeing Joan for some time since her divorce. She was an attractive and athletic 34-year-old.

> Oh, I never thought I would ever want a man again after Fred. Fred was so critical. He was always unhappy with me. I didn't clean the house right, dinner was late, or I was too fat. Nothing I did pleased him. He hated me. He hated his female boss. Apparently, his mother was the only woman he even halfway liked. And he was mad at her most of the time.
>
> I thought that I had learned my lesson about men with Fred until Tom came along. Tom seems to like everything I do. At first, I was suspicious. But we've known each other for 8 months now. Tom is so easy going. He is so uncritical and accepting of everybody. I feel so valued when I'm with him. And suddenly, I'm really horny. I never felt this way. Not even when I first dated Fred. This is a whole new thing for me, and I don't know what to make of it.

If Joan understood how oxytocin worked, she would know what to make of it. OXY seems to engender socio-sexual urges in animals and humans (Moore, 1987). It is centrally associated with maternal behavior and nurturance (Insel, 1992; Panksepp, 1992). It increases sexual desire in both males and females (Richard, Moos, & Freund-Mercier, 1991). But it seems particularly powerful in enhancing female sexual receptivity (Benelli, et al., 1994; Caldwell, et al., 1994). It can facilitate pair bonding and monogamy. Individuals prefer whom they are with when OXY increases (Carter, 1996). OXY is a prime candidate for mediating feelings of acceptance and social bonding (Panksepp, 1993). Carrying the theory a step further, Panksepp (1993) nominated OXY as a potential source of controlling child abuse and reducing the incidence of certain forms of impotence.

A synthetic version of OXY called pitocin is used to induce labor. Who knows? It might also some day become a female version of Viagra™. I am sure, however that Tom has facilitated its release in Joan's brain. OXY is primarily a female hormone.

Vasopressin (VP)

Al was a 58-year-old attorney whom I knew casually through my wife Marietta, a judge. I sometimes accompany her to law-related parties. At one occasion, Al cornered me in the bar. He had already consumed more than his legal limit when he offered me some background, followed by an important question:

> I was a hell of a stud when I was a young man, and I mean that in every sense of the word. I would hit on women, tell them I wanted a piece, and most of the time I would get slapped. But every now and again, I would get lucky. I was eager for a fight. I believed I was tougher than any man alive, and I was always ready to prove it. As a young lawyer, I loved a good yelling and shouting trial. I didn't want my cases to settle.
>
> I'm not like that now. I'm too old for bar fights. I will settle a case if I can avoid a court battle. I don't mind that so much. Probably it's better to be more peaceable. But I miss all the sexual piss and vinegar I had as a young man. I don't even chase my wife around the bed anymore. I even get offended at dirty jokes. Doc, I don't know what's happened to me. Can you tell me?

Yes, I could tell Al, but I didn't. Al is running out of the peptide vasopressin. In addition to restricting fluid output from the kidneys, VP raises the blood pressure. While it does not affect female socio-sexual behaviors, VP is especially effective with males. It turns them on sexually, and it raises their temper. VP promotes intra-species aggression, perhaps acting through the central amygdala. It is associated positively with levels of testosterone and estrogen. Panksepp (1993) believed that VP might be "a specific carrier for male dominance and persistence urges" (p. 94) and might promote heightened tendencies for males to exhibit aggression. Possibly, he argued, the underlying subjective emotional correlate of VP is one of increased irritability and anger.

Al's edges have softened because, as we age, we lose VP (Buck, 1999). Aging with its consequent loss of VP has a hand in mellowing men. VP is primarily a male hormone.

Gonadotropin-Releasing Hormone (GnRH)

Carla and Fred had been trying to have a baby for some time, with no results. They were consulting me because of the friction this was causing in their relationship. Carla spoke about this.

"Part of the problem was that we weren't doing it enough. And part of the problem, our doctor said, was that I didn't have enough follicles, or something like that."

"I'm not sure how I was involved in this," Fred said. "The doctor said my sperm count was low, and maybe my sperm were dull. Their pointy-ends were not sharp enough to stick them to the egg."

"So they gave us this gonad drug hormone," Carla explained. "And we are doing it. We do it in the morning, on the desk at noon, at bedtime, and when I have to wake up to pee. It's great. I will be sorry when I get pregnant and we don't get to take it anymore."

"Both of you take this drug?" I asked.

"Yes," they answered.

"Why?"

The answer, I found out, is that GnRH prepares females for ovulation and promotes spermatogenesis in males. GnRH functions by supporting the follicle-stimulating hormone (FSH). In 1993, Panksepp stated that GnRH "may well prove to be a prime mover in human libido" (p. 94).

That's why.

Corticotropin-Releasing Factor (CRF)

I was supervising Carol, a therapist, with 5 years in practice. She was discussing her work with Sarah, an abused client.

> We make progress, and then she does something to undo it. She cuts herself, or she binges and purges. She comes to see me, angry, blaming it on me. Then she will cry, apologize, beg me not to give up on her. For a week or so, she will do well, then she will decompensate. I've made

some progress. The suicidal gestures have stopped. It's like she can go so far, and then she hits a wall. I just don't get it.

If Carol knew about the corticotrophin-releasing factor (CRF), she would understand. It has very little to do with her work. A history of abuse can create "semi-permanent brain changes that at the psychological level may be experienced as (chronic) despair" (Panksepp, 1993, p. 92). CRF promotes fear and anxiety. Luckily, our brain has its own way of turning off CRF, and that is with norepinephrine (NE). The presence of CRF in the brain stimulates the release of NE in the brain. Thus, CRF creates its own demise by stimulating the release of NE. A serious problem can develop when stress becomes so chronic that CRF continues to be present in the brain. When this happens, supplies of NE are depleted, leaving nothing to contain or diminish the levels of CRF in the brain. With NE gone, there is no way to turn off the CRF. The brain is stuck in vigilance and fear.

Together with the neuromodulators, glucocorticoid (CRF) can cause permanent brain damage to the hippocampus. These neuromodulators can cause the neurons of the hippocampus to atrophy (McEwen & Sapolsky, 1995).

Carol must be patient with Sarah. Her job is to help Sarah stop catastrophizing and overreacting, create one safe place—Carol's office—and help Sarah build security, using Carol as a base. This will take time and patience on both Carol's and Sarah's parts. But most important, it will take commitment from them. When funds for the managed- care sessions run out, Carol will have to stay in there, working only for the co-pay or sometimes for free. And Sarah will have to endure the feeling of being given something.

Occasionally on my way home from the office, I ride by the housing projects. In Nashville, these apartments are sometimes behind a wall or a 6-foot fence, physically separating two worlds. I imagine the housing project life to be chaotic, violent, full of drugs, alcohol, and gunshots. I can only wonder if that is not what hell is. The norepinephrine amines of the children and their parents are depleted, and CRF is left in the brain to create fear on top of fear. I think of the neurochemical researchers, observing this same biochemical class dichotomy. I imagine them saying to themselves, "Some day we will make enough NE amines. Then, we can replenish the brain supply for all those who live in such a frightening, violent world. And this will cure our social ills."

I hope that is true. But I'm not a neurochemist. I am a therapist and, as such, am part priest, shaman, and scientist. I use faith, placebo, transitional objects, and social science. I am in search of a magic that is part spirit, intelligence, and courage. I believe we therapists can find that magic. I do not believe drugs will ever fix the human predicament of yearning or the pain that is part of growth. I still think we therapists, rabbis, and priests will always have a job, no matter what drugs are discovered.

The Emotion Neurocircuitry

Our brains are evolutionarily layered. Each layer adds emotional differentiation to its predecessor. The human brain has experienced three emotional evolutionary levels. In the brain's emotional neurocircuitry, these levels are represented by the brainstem/midbrain, the hypothalamus, and the limbic system (Buck, 1999). Each structure is replicated in each hemisphere, the right hemisphere and the left hemisphere. Emotions tend to have a specific base in one hemisphere or the other. In Wendy Heller's (1993) opinion, most are in the right hemisphere.

The Brainstem

My wife, my dog, Greco, and I were staying in a time-share vacation condo on the beach in Destin, Florida. It was 7 a.m. Day was breaking. I opened one eye to look at the ocean. Greco was restless and walking around sniffing, signaling he needed to go outside. I spied a lizard crawling down our screen door to the patio, perhaps stalking that nearby spider that was busily rebuilding its web. Suddenly, an alarm went off. I froze—and so did Greco, the lizard, and the spider. All were simultaneously paralyzed by the sound.

"What was that?" Marietta asked the question that Greco, the lizard, the spider, and I were asking, as she awoke.

Soon we would find out. Smoke from the air vents began to pour into our apartment. Greco raced to the back exit toward the beach. The lizard scrambled from the heat and smoke. I'm not sure what happened to the spider. But Marietta, Greco, and I quickly got the hell out of there.

The brainstem and midbrain mediate two survival functions. One is arousal/wakeful attention that, at its extreme, is the surprise (startle) response. This is what the dog, the lizard, and the humans in this apartment all participated in: We were startled together. Our brainstems and midbrain behaved exactly alike. Marietta voiced our common question, "What was that?"

Then, our primitive brains worked again in concert to avoid the danger of a fire.

The end of the story was that the next-door apartment had caught fire from faulty wiring in the air-conditioning system, causing the alarm and the sprinkler system to come on and extinguish the fire. We were settled back into our condo by the afternoon.

In the case of the brainstem, a network of fibers and cell bodies extends from the spinal cord to the thalamus. This is called the reticular formation

(Bremer, 1935). It produces electroencephalographic arousal and alerting and is the basis for general physiological arousal. As a system, this is called the ascending reticular activating system (ARAS) (Lindsley, 1957).

Apparently, this system is involved in two types of arousal activities. One is the startle response. The startle response can cause vocalization (as in Marietta's "What was that?"), urination, defecation, or ejaculation. This is a cholinergic response, using acetylcholine (ACH) as the neurotransmitter (Napier, Kalivas, & Hanin, 1991).

The second function controls approach and avoidance systems. This function has its origins in the limbic, midbrain area. Reward and punishment is the operative polarity here. Reward is centered in the medial forebrain bundle (MFB), and punishment is associated with the periventricular system (PVS). The endorphins (specifically substance P) are the neurotransmitters that carry the pain signal, while other endorphins carry the pleasure signal (LeGros, et al., 1938). Perhaps the spider and the lizard did not have this part of a neurological avoidance system.

One of the major functions of the brainstem is to manage the body's homeostasis. It acts as a stimuli filter. Stimuli that are constant, weak, or rhythmically repetitive are ignored or filtered out of our consciousness. We are programmed to attend to the unusual, the "what-is-wrong." We ignore our left ankle that is working well and instead attend to the unusual sensations coming from our sprained right ankle. Repetitive weak noises, like the sound of our mother's heartbeat while we are in the womb, might, in fact, relax and calm us. We will discuss this later in chapter 12 on sleep/fatigue/trance.

These neurostructures and neuromodulators worked to get us (dog, humans, perhaps lizards, and I don't know about the spider) safely out of that building.

The Hypothalamus

Remember Carla and Fred who were taking gonadotropin-releasing hormone (GnRH) to help them become fertile? Fred was telling of the day they successfully conceived.

> It was a strange day. Everywhere I went, I saw pregnant women. It made me mad to see all that fertility that I wanted so badly for us. I saw mating dogs stuck together, not being able to avoid successful procreation. I saw dragonflies doing it. Squirrels in the trees were going at it. Pigeons were fighting each other for the fertile female. On my way home for lunch, Carla called my cell phone to tell me that the thermometer indicated she was ovulating. By God, I would have killed any man who tried to get to my wife before I did. I walked in the door, picked Carla up, and

carried her straight to the bedroom. I meant business. I wouldn't say I was the best lover in the world that day, but I got the job done.

The hypothalamus is the next evolutionary brain level. It is involved in the reward-punishment system along with the brainstem and midbrain and in defense-and-attack systems, as well as sex, attachment, and submission. The hypothalamus, with its central location in the brain, is heavily supplied with blood vessels. This blood-supply system also transports chemicals that disclose the body's relative levels of fluids and hormones, as well as information relevant to nutrition (Hess, 1957).

The main function of the hypothalamus, given its critical location and supply of information and blood, is to control the autonomic nervous system (ANS). The parasympathetic system is one half of the ANS and governs rest, relaxation, submission, and attachment. Sex in the body is associated with the anterior hypothalamus. The sympathetic system (the other half of the ANS) governs the individual survival systems of aggression and fight/flight (Adams, 1979). The hypothalamus also controls the endocrine system in the body through the pituitary gland that is connected to the ventromedial region of the hypothalamus (Robertson & Sawyer, 1957; Rogers, 1954).

Even though it plays a central role in the brain, the hypothalamus does not directly influence emotions. Higher systems in the brain fulfill that function. But the hypothalamus does control the appetites—hunger, thirst, temperature balance, and sexual desire—and these have a great deal to do with our emotions.

The amygdala is an almond-shaped and sized part of the hypothalamus. We know the amygdala plays a principal role in the defensive red-alert fight/flight system in the brain (MacLean, 1993). What is not so well known is that an offensive attack of the predator is associated with another part of the brain. An offensive attack might have the same angry facial expression as a defensive one, teeth exposed and low-pitched threatening noises. But in the brain, the source of the defensive fear-induced attacks is located in the amygdala. The chase, consummatory, "I-want-that" attacks are centered in the lateral nucleus of the hypothalamus, the region associated with appetite.

The hypothalamus is important to the attachment-bonding process, related primarily to the distress calls of sadness and grief when mother and infant are separated. Pankseep (1981, 1982) found that these calls were highly associated with the brain's endogenous opiates, the endorphins. Endorphin centers in the hypothalamus are found in the anterior regions and the preoptic areas. Here, mammalian brains are distinguished from reptilian brains: Reptiles are born relatively self-sufficient and don't need tending from parents. Consequently, they do not have this brain apparatus for expressing sadness and grief at loss (Panksepp, 1982; Panksepp, Nelson, & Bekkedal,

1997). Sadness lowers our metabolic rate, and this may aid our survival as a species since we are not self-sufficient at birth.

As I mentioned, the hypothalamus controls all bodily appetites including sex. The ventromedial hypothalamus (VM) is the central-control site of the sex appetite. The VM is directly connected to the pituitary gland. When the sexual arousal signal comes from the VM, the pituitary gland releases a group of hormones into the bloodstream; chief among them is the gonadotropin-releasing hormone (Roberston & Sawyer, 1957; Rogers, 1954).

Two areas in the VM hypothalamus are particularly relevant. The lateral preoptic area (LPOA), when stimulated, produces exaggerated male sexual behavior in male rats. The medial preoptic area (MPOA) seems to have a greater relevance to female sexuality and maternal urges (Fisher, 1964). The anterior hypothalamus is the seat of this neural activity (Sawyer, 1969). Stimulation of this area increased male-like, sexual-imitating behavior in both males and females, for example, repeated mounting and thrusting. In addition to repeated mounting, males had continuous erections and shorter recovery periods following ejaculations (Vaughan & Fisher, 1962). Recent evidence suggests that the mating-induced activation system includes the medial preoptic areas of the hypothalamus, the amygdala, and the bed nucleus of the strea terminalis (BNST) (Newman, Parfitt, & Kollack-Walker, 1997). The MPOA has connectors to the ventral-tegmental area (VTA) in the midbrain. This promotes the opiate dopamine reward systems (Numan, 1996). The MPOA also projects into the septal area, turning on the more general appetites and the dopamine appetite reward systems as well (Panksepp, 1981).

The hypothalamus level of the brain—the emotion initiator—is more evolved and hence more a part of emotions. The higher the brain system, the more involved it is in emotions, emotional expression, and emotional awareness. The hypothalamus and the brainstem have more to do with drives and compulsions (Papez, 1937). Certainly, the hypothalamus was involved in Fred's lunchtime drive to impregnate Carla on the day they conceived.

Many emotion theorists do not see the drive/appetite system (the libido) as an emotion. I do. The libido is central to motivating and expressing desire, and it provides the internal push that may eventually lead to joy, the destination emotion. Heretofore, the part of the brain we have discussed comprises the reptilian brain. Reptiles have compulsions, but they do not have regrets or pride. That comes from the next evolution of the brain—the limbic system.

The Limbic System

Don was divorcing, and he was consulting me, hoping that I could help him cope with this difficult life challenge. A tornado raged through Nashville on

April 16, 1998. Don came to see me the day after the tornado. Here is what he told me:

> I used to live in East Nashville where the tornado hit. My children and their mother still do. When the tornado hit, I was stunned, frantic, helpless. I wasn't supposed to place calls to my ex-wife's house. But my children live there, too. I was scared. I was disgusted at myself and this divorce, that I was in a place where I could not take care of my children when they were threatened. I longed to see my children safe. I was ashamed. I didn't know what to do. I called anyway. No one answered.
>
> I drove over there. Trees were down everywhere. Some houses were gone. Others just damaged. Roads were blocked. Somehow I wound around the streets through the trees down and got to my old house. It was still standing. No damage. Down the street was my teenage daughter. I ran to her. We hugged. I was so happy. I don't think I have ever been so happy.
>
> Then, I was furious. How come my wife can have her family, and I am forced to abandon mine? If she were dead, they would live with me. I wanted her dead in that moment. And then I realized what I was wanting. I felt disgusted, and again I was sad. Suddenly, I was very tired. Once I found out everybody was all right, I went to my apartment and straight to bed. I slept for 10 hours.

In that space of 2 hours, Don experienced the nine human emotions that I consider basic emotions. They are all centered in the limbic system. This system completes the paleomammalian brain. According to P.D. MacLean (1993), its distinct parts are three to five layers of paleocortical tissue. No other part of the brain exerts so much impact on emotions.

A great deal of controversy focuses on what constitutes the limbic system. In 1996, Joseph LeDoux stated that parts of the limbic system serve functions having nothing to do with emotions and that all parts of the brain serve emotions in some way. But there remains no doubt that the area of the brain positioned between the hypothalamus and the neocortex—called the limbic system by some—is essential to the experience of emotion. Yes, of course, the amygdala (which is part of the hypothalamus, which is part of the limbic system) is intimately involved in emotional expression. And, yes, higher brain centers in the neocortex also are involved in emotional expression and awareness.

According to Ross Buck (1999), LeDoux (1996) correctly pronounced the end to considering the limbic system as the only source of emotional stimuli and added that previous discussions of the limbic system as a self-contained unit in this way were in error. Nonetheless, they contend that we still need a vehicle to discuss the emotional functions of this part of the brain, even if it has become somewhat of a metaphor rather than a concrete, specified reality.

There are three primary circuits in the limbic system (Pikaenen, Savander, & Le Doux, 1997). One is a circuit that connects the limbic system with the amygdala in the hypothalamus. This neurological wiring has to do with self-preservation, fighting, fear, and feeding. The second circuit is primarily identified with the septal area. It controls social sexual behaviors. The olfactory system is interconnected with both of these systems, while it bypasses the next circuit.

This third connector is the thalamocingulate circuit. It includes the mammal thalamic tract that connects mammillary bodies with the anterior thalamus through fibers extending to the cingulate gyrus. This circuit is associated with parental care and nursing, audiovocal communication to protect and nurture the young, and play behaviors.

As Don responded emotionally to the tornado, he did not know or care about the limbic system. He didn't care whether the limbic system was real or metaphoric. He didn't know about the three circuits that connect all the system's parts. They would only be relevant to him if some part of this system was not working. Then he would consult an expert, probably a neurologist, probably not a therapist. But it does no harm for a psychotherapist to know, for example, that the septal area of the brain controls social sexual behaviors.

In this chapter, I presented and briefly described some emotions involving neuromodulators and neurocircuitry. The purpose of this chapter was to introduce psychotherapists to the language of neuroscience and to help them put names to the neurological structures that support the emotional experiences they see every day in their offices.

Introduction to Chapters 5 through 14

Chapters 5 through 14 are organized similarly. Each chapter is about a neurologically mediated emotional experience. Chapters 5 through 13 each are about one discrete emotion. Chapter 14 is about empathy. Each chapter begins with a definition followed by a semi-fictional clinical case study, written as a story. This is followed by a neurological description of what is happening in the brain during the experience of the emotion that is the focus of the chapter. I then describe the physiology of the emotion. That is followed by a description of the positive strengths of the emotions and the negative consequences of the emotion. An examination of special aspects and problems of each emotion follows.

The chapter ends with the nomination of a ritual that might be helpful in moving clients out of an overdependence on that particular emotion and helping clients expand their emotional repertoire and move them into a positive healthy emotional flow. The ritual is followed by a concluding clinical case study, using the same characters demonstrating how the ritual can be effectively used.

After reading each of these chapters, the reader should know more about how the subject emotion works, its strength and weaknesses; how to help the client move out of the pathology of that emotion; and how to develop a ritual as a resource to help the client move from pathology to health.

CHAPTER **5**

Anger
The Most Dangerous Emotion

Anger Defined

While there is one facial expression of anger, anger can have two different adaptive functions, represented in separate neurological structures. The first and most recognized function of anger is defensive, a response to threat or to danger. The second is the consummatory anger of the predator. The facial expressions, the loud voice, the bared teeth, and the clenched fist all say, "I'm ready for a fight, so stop and submit" (Tomkins, 1963; Greenberg & Safran, 1986; Izard, 1971).

Defensive anger allows the object of the anger to withdraw. The predator's angry expressions are merely the first part of an attack. Played out this way, anger expresses dominance. It says, "You might as well submit, because I'm going to have my way."

Anger motivates and always provides energy. As a defense, anger is part of the amygdala system's red-alert fight/flight response (Adams, 1979). Anger prepares us for a defensive fight, which, of course, can quickly transform into a predatory offensive attack, where no prisoners are taken and dominance and consumption becomes the purpose.

Clinical Case Study

I was codirector of Compose, a program to prevent domestic violence. Most of our clients were court-ordered. John and Marsha were a couple participating in our program. Both were court-ordered. John explained:

"Before we came here, it was real bad. We would be talking, then suddenly we would be yelling. Sometimes I would push her."

"Or hit me," Marsha interjected.

"Yes, and sometimes it was her that hit me. One time, she came after me with a knife. I left, got in my car, and drove off. She got in hers and followed me. Before I knew it, she was driving beside me, her window down, cursing me, banging into the side of my car with hers. I punched the accelerator to get away from her, but she was right behind me. We were going 100 mph plus, weaving around cars. I was scared something bad would happen, so I got in the right lane. I let her get up close beside me on my left. As we were about to pass an exit and before she could ram me, I suddenly turned the steering wheel right. I about rolled the car. But I made it off the exit, and she kept on going down the Interstate. Our cars were banged up. Some door handles were gone. I went home, shaking. Marsha came home soon after that. We didn't talk for the rest of the day."

"Anger seems to ambush us," Marsha said. "It just comes up suddenly and takes us by surprise. We become stupid in less than 2 seconds."

The Neurology of Anger

Anger can follow two paths in the brain in order to put this emotion into action.

The first has to do with the thalamus-amygdala system. It is several synapses shorter than the second path that goes to the neocortex via the limbic system. The first quick path is the route of red-alert defensive anger.

The second path is longer and more cerebral in nature. Indeed, anger as an offensive attack is a complex emotional response, according to Gray (1977). Anger expressed this way is more considered, more calculated. It can be a decision to attack rather than a reflex to defend. In this second path, a larger brain circuit, the appetite circuitry, provides much of the neurocircuitry for anger. This includes the rest of the hypothalamus and the limbic system, as well as the neocortex. The neurohormones that are present in anger act as stimulants, giving power and energy to the whole body, while providing opiates to keep pain from affecting performance. Endorphin B and norepinephrine (NE) reduce pain. Vasopressin (VP) raises the blood pressure and increases heart rate (Koolhaas, et al., 1990).

Intelligence and Anger

Anger, especially defensive anger, shuts down the transmission of information from other parts of the brain. Endorphins render the neocortex inoperative. Our brains, therefore, are reduced to the paleomammalian brain, which is about the size of our fist. This part of our brain is fully mature by the age of 5, while the neocortex is not fully developed until age 26, (Panksepp, 1986).

Anger shuts down sensory input. We accept no information that does not support our reasons to be angry. Angry people rarely perceive reality as it is. They omit facts that don't support their anger. They use high-risk/reward, decision-making strategies that often result in poor decisions (Baumeister, Smart, & Boden, 1996).

Anger is full of cognitive distortions, particularly dichotomous thinking. Without the neocortex and with only the small mammalian brain, we cannot process complex thoughts. In red-alert situations, vigilant responses need to be immediate. Excess consideration would be dangerous. Doubt and second thoughts could get us killed. Therefore, we think in only two polarities: enemy/ally, good/bad, black/white, and so forth. Not only does anger filter out unwelcome information, it restricts our ability to think deeply.

Offensive anger is more complex and can include cunning and intelligent predatory planning. Still, dichotomous thinking dominates, and we filter out painful stimuli. Our intelligence remains compromised by this form of anger as well.

The Physiology of Anger

Anger increases the heart rate. It pulls blood toward the bone and away from the skin to protect the body from bleeding to death when injured. It increases blood pressure. It dilates the eyes and increases our food digestion to get rid of food so our bodies are filled with energy. It provides a keen focus and sense of purpose.

Anger is associated with many physical problems. Chronic anger negatively impacts the immune system. Angry people are frequently ill. Anger is particularly associated with hypertension, coronary-artery disease (Siegman & Smith 1994), and alcohol and drug abuse (Allan & Scheidt 1996).

The Negative Consequences of Anger

In addition to the physical problems anger can cause, it is easy to see the psychological damage, not to speak of the social pain, anger can cause. Anger is singularly the most socially controlled emotion. In order to deal with anger, police departments, courts, and prisons employ millions of people. No other emotional behavior receives such legislative attention, nor is any emotion more frequently spoken of from the pulpit.

Anger causes violence in families. It creates fear in others, destroying the social fabric of families and friendships. It creates paranoia and the impetus for delusional thinking, as we construct the justifications used to excuse anger.

Although it can certainly become an expression of insanity, the worst thing about anger is not so much that it makes us crazy, but that it makes us stupid. It also inhibits us from realizing how stupid we have become because of the justifications that follow.

"I wouldn't have hit her, if dinner had been ready. She deserved it." This is the second worst thing about anger: It creates righteous indignation and a sense of entitlement, where no justification or righteousness exists.

The Positive Consequences of Anger

Anger creates energy and a sense of purpose. It protects us from pain and powerfully focuses our attention. Angry people are often very successful. Tennis great John McEnroe is a celebrated example of a man who used anger as a powerful motivating force in competition. How many athletes have played without pain during a game, only to find out after the game that they were playing with a broken bone?

Anger helps us get things done. It speeds up our thinking. It gives us a sense that we are right. Confidence and focus come with this sense of purpose. Self-esteem is a part of anger. We feel entitled to our anger. It is here because we must right some wrong. We must do something. As an example, we know of angry people who have picked up automobiles to release people lying under the tires. Anger has been a powerful force in righting social wrongs in the American Revolution, the abolitionist movement, desegregation, and equal rights for women.

Anger comes from caring deeply and passionately about something. We would never be angry if we didn't desire something that we were frustrated by not having, or if we weren't protecting ourselves and those we love from some potential loss.

In a way, predatory anger is a compliment. It means that the object of this obsession is wanted and desired. Many people want to be the prey for a particular person's desire. When this works for the predator and the object of the predator's desire, some call this love, magic, or romance. Certainly, both parties are fortunate that one has the desire for the other and that the other wants to be the object of that intense passion. But there are times when the object of this passion does not wish for this attention. Then, predatory anger is at least intrusive and at worst dangerous.

Resolving Anger

Each emotion can resolve every other emotion, but the resolve might not be a healthy one. Let's consider each emotion, one at a time, as a potential candidate to resolve anger.

Fear can resolve anger. Children's anger is often resolved by the fear of a parent's disapproval. Resolving anger with fear only represses the anger and creates a feeling of cowardice. Also, fear is rarely a choice one can make coming from anger. If we assume that the amygdala mediates the fight/flight response in an emergency, if we assume anger is the fight half, and if we are thrown by the amygdala into anger, it is not easy for us to return voluntarily to fear. To resolve an emotion, we need a path that we can choose, and fear is not an easy choice from anger. And if, for example, a parent frightens a child out of anger and into fear, the consequences are usually shame and cowardice. Fear is rarely a positive resolve for anger.

Let's save *sadness* for the last emotion we nominate as the emotion to resolve anger and get us back into the flow.

Next, consider *joy*. Of course, when anger achieves a goal, joy resolves anger in the victory. If the victory is truly a reasonable achievement, the anger was justified, and joy is a healthy move from anger. But many times the victory and joy that can come from anger only perpetuate tyranny, and joy becomes an unhealthy resolution to anger.

Shame is an obvious resolve to anger. The problem is that shame is often toxic and, with toxicity still a part of shame, it will only create more hurt, which requires anger as a defense again. This is the typical batterer emotional cycle: anger → shame → anger → shame, and so forth. Shame, then, becomes the precursor to anger, not its resolution.

Interest/excitement/desire transforms anger from a defensive emotion into an offensive one. Becoming a predator is not necessarily bad, but we should not encourage it in a ritual, as it might create a painful legacy.

Surprise is a neutral emotion. It will take us out of anger, but no one knows where it will go from there.

Fatigue/rest/trance/sleep never harmed an angry person. These might provide moments of calm and peace, but all too often, once an angry person awakes from the trance, he or she might find anger again.

Disgust is an important cog in the CAD (contempt-anger-disgust) triad (Rozin, et al., 1999). But disgust adds fuel to anger and provides anger's justification. It does not resolve anger.

Treating Anger

Treating anger requires a carrot and stick. Fear will always overcome anger. The angry-confident person easily can flip the switch to the flight part of the fight/flight red-alert system in the brain. Similar brain circuitry is at work. Many neurohormones are shared. Though fear can be almost as stupid as anger, often it has a bit more intelligence.

Fear is the emotional base of respect. And an authority must have respect in order to be effective. Having a stick that creates fear and respect will stop anger quickly. Sometimes fear is an important treatment resource. Police and the courts can serve as the stick. Therapists and treatment programs can be the carrot. As I noted earlier, fear is a poor end-point for the journey out of anger, and we can rarely choose fear on our own. If we submit just because the other individual is dominant and we are afraid, we can hate ourselves and the other person. No real internal change occurs. When the source of fear leaves, the same behavior returns. This creates much shame and resentment.

Once our anger is contained for whatever reason, the next step is to help the angry person find a path to sadness. When we reach sadness, we will discover the intelligence embedded in that emotion. Sadness is a healthy path of resolve for anger. When the angry person lets go of her predatory goal and grieves the loss, the healthy resolution of anger is not far behind.

Steven Stosny founded the Compassion Program based on this premise. (We modeled our Nashville Compose Program after this.) Stosny treated sexually offending priests for the Catholic Church in the Catholic psychiatric hospital in Washington, D.C. In a visit to a Duluth-(Minnesota) model batterers program, he discovered why that model had been so ineffective in treating perpetrators of family violence. These programs treat anger with shame. At conventions of domestic violence counselors, defenders of the Duluth model declare that these men[5] are difficult, if not impossible, to treat. Incarceration is clearly the only option. This blames the batterer for the program's ineffectiveness, much like the batterer often blames the victim for the battering (Stosny 1995).

Stosny's premise was that anger is a defense against hurt. Shaming the batterer only creates more hurt. And, hence, more anger. This is why the Duluth model cannot accommodate couples and why battering often reoccurs in families when the program participant returns home after attending a Duluth-model program.

According to Adele Harrell (1991), Duluth-model participants are as likely or more likely to batter after completing the program than they were before treatment. This is the one place where therapy seems to break the Hippocratic oath "to do no harm."

In contrast, Stosny's Compassion Program graduated 75% of its participants, and 90% of its graduates did not re-offend for 1 year posttreatment. This contrasts with the Duluth model that graduates less than 50% and 90% of whose graduates re-offend within 1 year of treatment (Stosny, 1995).

In introducing his program, Stosny began by discussing his own violent father, whom he loved. According to Stosny, coping with anger is a universal problem that we all must master. And, of course, he stated that mastering our anger is not easy.

The Compassion Program was there not to condemn. It was there to teach skills, primarily the skill of focusing below the anger to feel the sadness and hurt first. Feeling sadness derails anger's momentum. Sadness pushes different neurohormones in the brain other than those associated with anger. It takes courage to give up the defense of anger and to feel sad and hurt. It is easier just to let the anger take over the brain.

Sadness neurohormones dissolve anger neurohormones. After focusing on the hurt that the anger defends, the next step is to contain shame and self-attacks by offering compassion to one's self. The final step is to learn perspective-taking and empathy by having respect and compassion for the person who was, at one time, the focus of the anger. This brings self-esteem and pride (joy) in one's own character—pride that we have the capacity to give compassion and understanding, even to an opponent. This last step focuses on the universal sadness and tragedy of the human experience and ends in the joy, self-esteem, and pride that are by-products of compassion.

Stosny calls the skill he teaches the HEALS technique. It is an acronym. I have adapted this technique and rewritten it for our Compose Program. My version is the HEART ritual:

 Step 1: Imagine seeing in flashing images before you, the letters <u>H</u> A L T or <u>H</u> E A R T. Focus on these to contain your anger. This step uses willpower, which only lasts about 40 seconds.

 Step 2: After you have contained your behavior, <u>E</u>xamine the hurt below the anger. Nominations for words that express your hurt and sadness are: unimportant; disregarded; valueless; accused; powerless or inadequate; unlovable or rejected; and disgusting or unfit for human contact. Choose one or more. Feel these feelings for about 20 seconds. This will put in your brain the real feelings of sadness that your anger protects you from feeling. This changes your neurohormones from anger neurohormones to brain chemicals that signal your body that you are sad.

 Step 3: Once you have realized that you felt unimportant, disregarded, unworthy, or valueless, and so forth. <u>A</u>sk the question of common sense. Is it true that at your core you are *unimportant or do not matter?* The answer is always NO! This inoculates you from toxic shame.

 Step 4: Now that you have reaffirmed your basic worth, look inside and give <u>R</u>espect to the other person or look inside them and see that what that person feels. Possibly, that person feels some of the same feelings that you do. He or she is most likely feeling one or more of these: unimportant; unworthy of regard; valueless;

accused; powerless or inadequate; unlovable or rejected; disgusting or unfit for human contact. This is a tragedy. You were hurt, and the other person perhaps still is hurt. Respect this person and his or her feelings. You are now sad for yourself and sad for your adversary, as well. In this state of respect, you are expressing compassion as well. The next step becomes easier after you have completed this one.

 Step 5: Together solve the problem, or wait until you can work together to solve the problem.

Step One, H, requires *self-control*, self-discipline, and willpower. To exercise this control, you must be aware of your emerging anger. Even if you feel out of control, you can achieve this level of awareness by recognizing your body's physical signs that indicate you are about to be angry. Is your heart racing? Are your teeth and fists clenched? Is your voice loud? Is your back tense? Willpower is important in any effort to change. But willpower by itself will work for only about 40 seconds. It is a way to prepare us to do something that will be more effective in managing our emotions. Too often we use *only* willpower, either because we don't know what else to do, or because we don't want to do anything else (especially to stop and feel the sadness in the hurt). Willpower—this first step—will get us started on the process of self-awareness and self-responsibility, but it won't get us all the way to our goal. To get closer to the goal, move to Step Two.

Step Two, E, requires self-awareness. What hurt are you defending with anger? How do you feel below your anger? After you have contained yourself, Examine the hurt feelings below the anger: "I am feeling . . ."

This emotion is *always* a sense of one of the following:

- Unimportant
- Disregarded
- Valueless
- Accused
- Powerless or inadequate
- Unlovable or rejected
- Disgusting or unfit for human contact

The temptation here is to hope Step One, self-control, will numb our feelings so we do not have to feel them. Step One alone is rarely enough. We need to feel and express what we feel. Once you have identified the hurt below the anger, remember another time, long ago, when you felt the same feelings. For 20 seconds, let yourself remember and feel those feelings. This takes courage. Sadness is usually a safe way to express a powerful feeling, but it is hard to do. Anger is easier.

Self-awareness is the base from which all personal growth and responsibility begins. If we are to change, we must feel our real feelings. We must have the courage to feel sad and face the loss. Feeling the sadness from a time long ago reminds us that we are not working on this situation that hurt us now. We are working on ourselves and transforming our anger to sadness. Labeling our feelings takes us out of the hypothalamus and engages the neocortex. This is the point at which the anger neurohormones are exchanged for the sadness neurohormones. (You can see when this happens because the participant's eyes often look downward.)

Step Three, A, requires a realization that the socialization process has lied to us about ourselves. These lies conclude that we are unimportant, worthy of disregard, valueless as a person, powerless or inadequate, unlovable, disgusting, or unfit for human contact.

Although we might know that these descriptions are lies, they still hurt us. When we fight others to protect ourselves from this hurt, we really are fighting years upon years of shame. It is like an electrical burn. On the outside, there appears to be no injury. But if someone touches the skin of a part of the body that has been electrically burned, a blister will appear. It will seem as if the touch caused the burn, but it didn't. The burn rose from deep under the skin. In this step, our job is to tell the truth about who we are at our core. We are valuable, important, lovable, powerful. These feelings protect us from the toxic shame that comes from an actual experience that is not now present. In Step Three, we are simply using *common sense* and telling the truth about who we are. We are at the core important, worthy, valuable, well-intended, powerful, lovable, and fit to be a good friend.

Step Four, R, requires we respect the other person and consider how that individual feels. In this step, we use the skill of *spiritual connectedness*. After we have defended and respected ourselves in Step Three, we are in a position to respect and love others. We ask ourselves if we know enough about the other person to know what he or she might be feeling. If we are having trouble figuring this out, a good guess is that this individual is feeling *the same hurt* we were feeling when we identified our hurt below our anger in Step Two.

Step Five, T, tells us to move forward, solve the problem. Sometimes we cannot find a collaborator in problem-solving. They may not trust us. Or, they may be trapped in their own anger. If we have reached this point, we have solved the problem of anger in us. This may be all we can do for now.

Working with a Chronically Angry Client

Often other people want to push their hurt on to us by passing the blame and shame they feel onto one of our many mistakes. If we accept the shame they give us and reinforce it with anger, we injure and re-injure each other.

In a relationship, when one partner stops this blame-shame-anger-hurt-blame cycle by containing his or her hurt, that person can begin the process of spiritual connecting, which is also called *love or compassion*. Anger leads to more anger, but compassion leads to more compassion—most of the time. Certainly, compassion will stop the anger cycle.

When treating a chronically angry person, placating anger only reinforces anger. Trying to help an angry person by giving into this individual will encourage an angry person to continue to escalate angry behavior. Anger can become an addiction. Anger creates an internal drug event. The drug event feels good and, in addition, other people often reinforce anger by giving into it. Like any addiction, treatment begins when someone hits a bottom. A bottom becomes a floor and the foundation for recovery. One hits a bottom when he or she sincerely says, "I will do whatever it takes to get better."

The stick in the form of the police, the courts, and the threat of jail can help create a bottom. With a bottom in place, giving compassion and teaching compassion in the form of the HEART ritual is an effective carrot with a stick.

Conclusion and Summary

On one hand, anger is an emotion associated with many bad things and a great deal of pain. On the other, anger can be an incredibly powerful force for change and success. If anger is one's primary emotional expression, the pathology will not only be a part of that angry person, but pathology also will be contagious. It will surround the angry person with fearful, shamed people. The people who are captive of the angry person will be filled with grief and pain, until that angry person meets someone or some situation that helps the angry person to begin anger's healthy resolution. Probably that someone appears in the form of a police person, not a therapist. If a therapist is asked to help, we hope that therapist will have something to offer, a carrot to the policeman's stick.

Clinical Case Study: Anger Resolved

For several weeks since John and Marsha told this story about the banging cars, I noticed that John was coming alone. After class one week, John waited to talk with me alone.

"Me and Marsha," he said, "we broke up."

"I'm sorry," I said. "I know you loved her."

"I did. I loved her, but you know, Doc, I think its better this way. I got control of my anger. I used that HEART meditation every day. I practiced and practiced it. I got good at it. I figured out I was not so angry as I was sad. And when I feel sad, I don't feel angry."

"That's great," I said.

"But Marsha, she couldn't do it. When I had compassion for her, it made her madder. She said I thought I was better than her. I didn't think that. I was proud that I wasn't angry no more, and I was sorry she still was. She didn't think she needed to practice HEART. After that time we tore off each other's door handles on the Interstate, I knew I had to get serious about this. So I worked on it, and she didn't."

"Changing old patterns in a relationship is hard," I said. "Changing an old pattern in yourself is tough enough, but you cannot change another person. Maybe it is better. Some couples seem to never be able to escape their past. It is better to break up than to break a bone or go to jail. It's sad. But with learning to control your anger, you can have a new healthy relationship."

On the last session, John brought his new girlfriend.

"I wanted you to meet Carla," John said, as he introduced me to her. "She's good for me."

"And he's good for me, too," Carla added. "John tells me that this class changed his life and that he is better for it. If that's true, I'm better for it too. Thank you, Doc."

CHAPTER **6**

Fear
The Most Avoidant Emotion

Fear Defined

Fear is the other half of the fight/flight response. It shares much of the brain chemicals and neurostructure of anger. Fear (along with disgust) is also on one polarity of the approach/avoidance structure (Rozin, Lowery, Imada, & Haidt, 1999). Fear can mean "flee," "run," "get out of here." But it can also mean "avoid," "go the other way," "hide," or "be still and maybe they won't notice."

Fear comes from a threat that is more powerful than we are. Fear announces that this threat might hurt us, either physically or emotionally. In fear, the face seems to freeze (Izard, 1971). The skin becomes cool, pale, and sweaty. Fear turns up the body heat, increases the heart rate and breathing. Fear amplifies attention, thinking, and access to memory. It creates so much mental activity that we become mentally paralyzed. Breath moves to the top of the lungs. Often, hyperventilation is the consequence. Memories of other frightening times flood the mind (Greenberg, 2001; Greenberg & Paivio, 1997).

On the other hand, healthy fear can protect us. Fear can help us be careful and cautious. Fear is associated with respect, sensitivity, kindness, and submission (Olds, 1977).

Clinical Case Study

I was seeing Anthony. A successful accountant, he was 32 and unmarried.

"I'm good at details," Anthony explained. "Somehow dealing with minutiae is comforting, the smaller the better. I like to clean house, too. You'd think I would find a woman who would appreciate that skill. If I could, I would spend my life cleaning house or auditing books for small businesses and preparing taxes. But I have to go to the grocery store. I have to meet clients. I am so anxious being with people that I can barely leave the house.

"My child psychologist told my mother that it began when I was 4. I had nephritis before they discovered a drug to treat it. My mother took me to the Mayo Clinic. They told her that I would die if I didn't eat, and I wasn't ever hungry. She put me in a chair. She sat across from me with food. I stubbornly refused to eat. Tears would come to her eyes. Then, her face would look real angry and determined, and she would slap me. I would cry, and when I opened my mouth, she would shove food into me. The doctors say that this saved my life. My child psychologist said that it made me chronically afraid.

"It's not my fault. It's not my mother's fault. It's just that way. I still have trouble trusting women, especially my mother. But I don't even trust my own brother, and my father's dead.

"Now, my boss wants me to fly with him to Chicago next month. I'm terrified of flying. I will quit my job first. If I can't control it, put it in a category, or clean it, I am afraid of it. And there is not much in this world I can control."

Neurology of Fear

Although fear has many neural-circuitry overlaps with anger (that is, both are centered in the amygdale; Morgan, Romanski, & LeDoux, 1993), some important differences exist (Fanselow, 1994).

Whereas the anger circuit is focused in the medial amygdala, fear is in the central and lateral amygdala. Anger utilizes the perifornical hypothalamus, while fear circuitry includes the medial hypothalamus. Both anger and fear extend to the dorsal periaqueductal gray (LeDoux, 1996; Maier, et al., 1993).

The anger neurohormones energize the body, anesthetize pain, and give confidence. Fear neurohormones also energize the body. Although they can sensitize us to pain (McGaugh, et al., 1995), they do not relieve pain. Fear hormones do not bring confidence with them. Rather, they bring doubt and confusion (Lang, Bradley, & Cuthburt, 1990). The fear neurohormones include many of the neuropeptides, for example, diazepan-binding inhibitor (DBI), and corticotropin-releasing factor (CRF), which is strongly associated with chronic trauma and child abuse. Associated with fear are cholecystokinin, CCK, alpha melancyte-stimulating hormone and neuropeptide Y, and glutamate (Panksepp, et al., 1991).

Fear and Intelligence

Fear makes us almost as stupid as anger, but not quite. Anger sends us boldly into action, albeit sometimes ill-considered action. Fear shrouds us in confusion, doubt, and uncertainty (Lang, et al., 1990). We are so flooded with stimuli and memories of previous painful times that we cannot think straight. The only good thing about this is that when we are afraid, we know that we aren't thinking straight. We believe we are in danger, and we hope to find a sanctuary soon. Along with the safety and the calm we seek, we hope our return to sanity will come as well.

The main effect that fear has on the brain is in our memory. Fear both dulls and sharpens our memories at the same time. Fear spreads our attention focus away from the object of threat, and we attend strongly to details of the context of the threat. In a car wreck we may not remember how it happened, but we may remember details that seem irrelevant, like the flowers by the side of the road. This is called flashbulb memory (LeDoux, 1996). This memory helps us debrief a traumatic event. We can pick from all the details of this picture in the brain and evaluate what is really relevant, when at the moment of trauma we do not have the time for such attention to detail.

While this helps us learn from our trauma, it also establishes the foundation for phobias. These irrelevant details can become associated with fear, so that when we see one of them again our fear response is triggered, when, in fact, there is no danger.

The Physiology of Fear

Fear covers more or less the same territory in the body as anger: increase in blood pressure and heart rate, gastric motility, and increase in body tension. But subtle differences exist. Blood pressure is higher in anger than in fear. Finger temperatures decrease less in fear than anger. This means that anger pushes more blood to the deep tissue near the bone than does fear. It also means that fear is more sensitive and aware than anger (Levenson, et al., 1990). In fear, hyperventilation occurs more often. In fear, the increase in heart rate is smaller. There are larger increases in cardiac output and stroke volume, smaller increases in facial temperature, and smaller increases in finger-pulse volume (Ekman, et al., 1983). From this data, we can conclude that fear acts more on the heart muscle, while anger acts more on the vasculature.

The Negative Consequences of Fear

Chronic fear eventually leads to depression and hopelessness. Being afraid means that you still have something to lose. Eventually, people can become tired of being afraid. The only way out of their fear is to give up caring, letting go of their stake in life. This becomes cynicism, chronic depression, and despair. (These characteristics will be elaborated on in chapter 7 on sadness).

Fear can create many of the same health problems as anger: an impaired immune system, heart problems, cancer, and so forth. These problems seem to be a little less severe in fear, perhaps because fear is not addictive while anger is. While many people enjoy confidence and dominance that comes along with anger, no one enjoys being afraid.

Fear can encourage addiction to drugs. Fear along with shame and sadness are the three main feelings that people try to escape by using crutches such as alcohol, heroin, benzodiazopines, cocaine, and marijuana. Many people would much prefer drugs to fear; for many, fear or drugs seem to be their only options.

Real fears can become compounded with imagined fears, both of which can be magnified by painful memories (Morgan & LeDoux, 1995). Fears, then, can take on lives of their own, with little reference to logic or reality.

This does not mean that the fears are not real. Phobias of things, people, and settings can emerge and grow. People can be trapped in their homes because of fear or forced to travel by a slower or more dangerous medium of transportation. For example, fear of airplanes forces us to travel by car or bus; fear of elevators forces us to take the stairs.

Positive Consequences of Fear

Success can be a consequence of fear. When we are afraid of failing, we plan. We practice. We prepare. And when it is our turn at bat, we hit the ball. We become a success because of all our hard work. That work was a consequence of fear.

Respect is a consequence of fear. Perhaps we need not fear poisonous snakes, guns, or chain saws. But it is important that we respect the dangers they pose. Respect is a product of fear with a bit of knowledge and wisdom added. We all need to look both ways before crossing a dangerous street. We all need to respect authority and the feelings of others. Caution and respect are healthy aspects of fear.

Some of us never get angry. We use fear instead. Although I don't recommend this emotional stance, along with it can come a kind, sensitive person who knows what it is like to be afraid. These people often help people who are afraid. They reassure strangers that they pose no threat. They help others who are frightened and disconnected, because they understand how they feel.

This kindness can come at great cost. Anger can be an important source of strength and energy. Giving it up and allowing fear to be our only response to danger is like losing an emotional right arm.

Catastrophizing

We all do this, some of us more than others. We worry about things that might or might not happen in the future. There are the famous catastrophizers who believe that the world is coming to an end. Others of us worry that our child, who is out riding a bike, will fall and break her neck.

Therapist Yvonne Agazarian[6] has a way of dealing with us worriers when we borrow fear from the future in this way. I learned this by attending one of her magnificent seminars. She says to the worrier, "You are at a fork in the road. And you have pushed yourself into the future beyond the fork, believing the worst. But really you are at a fork in the road, not in the future. Can you tell the future?" The worrier's obvious answer is "no."

"Well, since you cannot foresee the future," she continues, "and you really don't know what will happen, I want to invite you to consider coming back to that fork-in-the- road. Here, you are in the present and you can be curious about the future. Can you come back to not-knowing and wonder?"

When the answer is a sincere "yes," Yvonne often asks, "Which feels better, living in fear of a predicted future that you really can't predict, or living in the present, not knowing and wondering?"

Usually the answer is that it feels better living in the present, in the un-known, wondering, seeing potential good and bad outcomes, preparing for the bad, hoping for the good, and being curious to see how reality will play out in the future. Yvonne's cognitive behavioral technique for managing catastrophizing resolves fear with wonder. When she reminds the worrier that not knowing is a more accurate, honest statement, she invites the worrier to leave the hyped-up, vigilant brain chemistry of fear and to come back to neutral, to not-knowing, to what she calls "the fork in the road," where you don't know and you can wonder, imagining good possibilities as well as bad ones.

Surprise and Fear

Though wonder, the mild part of startle/surprise/wonder, helps resolve imagined fears borrowed from the future, the more intense startle/surprise emotion only embellishes our fears. The goal of fear is to motivate the person to withdraw, run away from, or avoid danger. It is the signal to retreat to safety. Safety means that you move toward a place where you know what to expect, where you have control over what will happen.

Surprise, even if it is intended to be positive, is not welcome in the context of fear. Rarely does surprise resolve fear. Fear arouses us; then surprise arouses us further into terror. When counseling a frightened person, we want to help her find as much certainty and control as possible. If, for example, you are driving a car with an adult passenger, and that adult is frightened by the traffic, stop and suggest that she might feel better if she drove. Once she gets behind the wheel, she will usually become calmer, because she feels a sense of control.

When a child is frightened, you can help her feel more in control by giving her choices: "Would you rather go with your mother or father?"; "Do you want to take along a toy?"; "What would you like to wear?" Choices give children and adults a sense of control and mastery. Control and predictability help calm fears.

Never say, "Relax, I will decide" or "Stop worrying, I will take care of it." These words only make the frightened child or adult feel out of control and more afraid. Almost always, people with a strong need for control use control to cover their fears.

Why Most Therapies Help Reduce Fear

Behaviorists and cognitive behaviorists have often criticized Rogerian and psychoanalytic therapy as being ineffective treatment and a waste of time and money. Research indicates that all therapeutic approaches can work if the client trusts and respects the therapist.

The reason traditional psychotherapy works with fear is because most of us are ashamed to admit we are afraid. The word coward comes quickly to our minds when we are afraid. We become afraid of being a coward. We try to stop being afraid, and that doesn't work. When we find a therapist who will accept our fears, we stop worrying about being a coward and start dealing with our fears. This allows us to express our fears freely without threat of shame. We then can begin to accept ourselves and sort through our fears, keeping those we need to keep and letting go of those that confine us. With this safe context, we can begin to take risks and face fears, and we are able to become more realistic about them. Our fears become smaller. Fear, in effect, begins to recede the minute we are no longer afraid of fear (Rutledge, 2003).

Other treatment approaches also are effective with treating fear-related problems, because once fear is faced and accepted, there are many ways to help reality seep into consciousness. The first step to treating fear is to embrace fear with your client.

Beginning to Help the Fearful Client

Never tell clients that their fears are crazy or unreasonable. Never ridicule or make fun of their fears. Fear is an instinctive response to danger. Sometimes we are afraid and do not know why. (Note that rape prevention classes teach women to honor their instinctive fears that might appear unreasonable.) When we feel our fears are unreasonable and perhaps evidence that we are crazy, we learn to hide our fears. After repressing our fear in this way inside we feel afraid, ashamed, and very alone.

Some people use blame, intimidation, and control to help them cope with their fears. Often it is the bully who is really afraid. People can be so ashamed of their frightening feelings that they cannot give them a name. As a therapist, the first thing we should do is to respect our clients. Let them know that whatever they are feeling, we can understand. Then we can help them identify their feelings so that they are comfortable sharing their fears with us. We hope that therapists are interested in how their clients really feel, that they will truly understand, and that clients won't be made to feel ashamed of what they feel.

Once clients are safe to feel and talk about feelings with their therapist, the second step for the therapist is to help these clients make sense of their fears. Fears may be a response to a dangerous situation. For example, when a frightened child races into the house screaming for help because a stranger in a raincoat tried to pull her into a car, there is no question that her fear propelled her into the safest and best course of action—to run away.

As an adult, that child might become frightened of men in raincoats and not really understand why. Our job as therapists is to help our clients connect dots like these. When people have a frame for their fears, their fears do not seem quite so large. They don't feel so crazy.

Cognitive Loops[7]

In our work, we often see clients who have problems with anxiety and find themselves stuck in patterns of rumination and constant worrying. These worried thinking patterns are called cognitive loops, because the thinking in our minds seems to go in circles, never really giving us a sense of direction.

There is a reason an individual becomes stuck in a cognitive loop when a course of action needs to be taken. Taking action always involves some risk, and we are afraid of risk. Though it is ultimately not in our best interests to become stuck in a cognitive loop, it does slow us down and seems to protect us from the risks involved in taking action. We might not be fully conscious of it, but the loop can give us a safe place to hide. The cognitive loop can provide considerable secondary gain. The problem, however, is that our life can come to a standstill, while we are trapped by our worries. The cognitive loop does not solve our real problems or the problems with our chronic anxiety that are the consequence of a cognitive loop.

How does an individual form a cognitive loop? The answer is by placing two positive values in opposition to each other. We can convince ourselves that our two values are in opposition to one another. Closer examination almost always reveals they are not opposed to each other at all. The loop helps us avoid taking a feared course of action. To keep us confused and in the loop, we must keep these values connected and in opposition to each other in our minds, trying to serve both values simultaneously. (The truth is all values that are good values will integrate, if we can creatively expand our options.)

When we are in a cognitive loop, we are stuck in our mammalian brain. Remember? This is the small, fist-sized part of the brain, just above the brain stem. This part of the brain confines us to two choices. In a cognitive loop, we give each choice equal weight, and thus we cannot move in either direction.

To escape this loop, we need access to our neocortex, the human brain, where we can call on creativity and come up with more choices. To get to our human brain and to access our creativity, we need to nominate a third position (Newbrough, 1995). Third position creates a tie-breaking vote. It shifts the balance in our mind toward a specific direction.

Suppose Sarah is trying to decide whether to travel out of town to spend the holidays with her parents, siblings, and in-laws, or to relax, stay at home to be with her husband and friends. Sarah has a history of conflict with certain family members and almost always becomes upset when visiting them. She believes going to the beach with her family would be more relaxing and enjoyable. On the other hand, she loves her family, including those with whom she has conflict, and she strongly believes in the importance of family and sharing in family traditions.

Sarah has put herself into a cognitive loop by placing her value that the holidays are a time of relaxation and enjoyment in opposition to her value of family. But are these values really as opposed to each other as she has convinced herself that they are? Is there a third position?

To get out of a cognitive loop, we take one value at a time and follow it to its logical outcome, without considering the other value. When we conclude our imaginary journey, pursuing our first value, we ask: Is the other value really in conflict with this one? If this process is followed honestly, the answer is almost always, "No, the values are not really opposed." We follow the same imaginary process with the second value and again inquire, "Are the values opposed?" If we have been honest in our inquiry, the answer is likely, "No."

There are two clear values. One is serving the self. A second value is duty to others, in this case, specifically, it is duty to family. Once the two values are clarified and disconnected we choose a third value, a third position. A third value might be Sarah's loyalty to her husband. What does he need from her?

With these values clarified and a third position chosen, the next step is to search for the secondary gain. Here, we wonder why we placed these values in opposition to one another. How would the paralysis of worry help us? Perhaps Sarah is serving what once was an invisible third value. Perhaps she is placing these values as mutually exclusive "either/ors," because she wants to protect her innocence. Sarah wants to be seen by her husband and others as a good person, a person who worries and wants to do the right thing.

As Sarah follows the value of using vacation for rest and renewal, she imagines herself on a beach, lying in the sun. She asks whether or not her family would object to that. The answer clearly is, "No."

Next, she imagines following the value of attending family rituals and traditions. She imagines herself at Thanksgiving dinner. She asks herself whether or not her beach-vacationing self would object, and the answer clearly is, "No."

Then, Sarah asks the question of her husband. What is the right thing to do by him? This is her third tie-breaking value. Her husband has no problem with her family. Going to visit relatives over the holiday is something he wants to do. He would also like her support to visit his family.

Now, Sarah wonders why she placed these values in conflict. What good would come of her worrying? The answer was clear: "It would help me avoid the conflict that happens when I go home." This is her secondary gain. That clearly was the problem that she needed to face. Her husband was not afraid; she was. How might she deal with the conflict that happens when she visits her family?

Almost always a cognitive loop creates an aura of innocence and good-ness around the worrier, protecting the worrier from shame and also from some important difficult action that resolving the cognitive loop would require. The third position gives us perspective and clarity. From Sarah's husband's point of view, it became obvious to her. The cognitive loop was undone.

We worriers reassure ourselves of our basic goodness when we surround ourselves with swirling righteous values. And are we not a good person for caring so deeply and worrying so intensely? But this truth usually is that we are not quite so good. We are afraid of facing something that we, somewhere inside ourselves, know we need to face.

This process unraveled Sarah's cognitive loop and gave her a sense of direction. She can now plan to visit her family for part of the holiday and address her conflict. She can leave her family and spend the remaining time on the beach, relaxing with her husband.

Once the secondary gain is discovered, we need to use the CALMS meditation, described later in this chapter, to help us face our real fear, the fear that was the driving force in creating our cognitive loop.

If she had not resolved this obsessive worry, she might have avoided the family visit and achieved her goal of using the time to relax by going to the beach. But while there, she would protect her innocence by feeling guilty the whole time worrying about not visiting her family. While this would help her avoid her family conflict, her decision only extends the worry and adds somatic misery to her emotional anguish. When she visits her family instead, this resolution will help her negotiate an effective peace with her estranged siblings and parents—or help her develop necessary effective defenses that she dreads putting in place.

The Construction of a Phobia

Phobias come from avoiding the context of a past trauma. They are established with the details of flashbulb memory (LeDoux, 1996). Rumination on the details from the flashbulb contextual memory can refire the amygdala. For example, perhaps you were in a car wreck and your memory captured the image of daffodils at the scene of the wreck. When you recall the wreck, your fear response is triggered. As you ruminate about the wreck, with fear taking over your mind and body, you keep seeing in your mind's eye daffodils. Daffodils become associated with fear. The association is further solidified each time you remember the car wreck. In the brain, what is wired together fires together. Eventually, just seeing daffodils can trigger your fear response. Once solidified in this way, a person may avoid going outside during the month when daffodils bloom.

The brain is wired so that there are extensive connections from the amygdala to the neocortex to tell the reasoning part of the brain to be afraid. Very few connections come back from the neocortex to the amygdala to tell the fear response that, reasonably, there is nothing to fear (LeDoux, 1996). Therefore it is difficult for us to try to tell ourselves not to be afraid. As I am sure you know, often telling someone that there is no reason to be afraid does not work. Because fear is so difficult to control, often Beta-blockers are prescribed to prevent the constant trauma phobic response. Beta-blockers turn down the sympathetic nervous system (Johnson, 2004), and this makes the amygdala less likely to fire.

Obsessive-Compulsive Disorder (OCD)

This is a fear-based emotional knot. Just as a pacifier calms an infant, just as a blankie calms a toddler, and a favorite stuffed animal calms a child, repetitive ritualistic behaviors can calm adult fears. Because rituals work to calm fears (the basis on of this book), these behaviors become entrenched. OCD is similar to a phobia. Remember, avoiding a fear stimulus increases a phobia. Repeating a ritual to avoid a calamity increases the obsession with the fear and OCD ritual.

With OCD when the brain confronts fear, it locks on to fear like a sticky transmission in a car and won't let go until the ritual releases it. Often, rituals don't work, but it is the random reinforcement of the ritual working sometimes that keeps this behavior in place. Remember Jeffrey Schwartz (2004) from chapter 3? He studied neurological functioning with OCD patients. He found a brain circuit that is particularly indicated here. The three parts of the circuit are the caudate nucleus (a part of the striatum), the orbital frontal cortex, and the anterior cingulate gyrus.

Normally, the striatum (and its caudate nucleus) work as a gatekeeper, sorting information and encouraging its flow through the brain. But in OCD patients, the caudate nucleus gets stuck when fear comes, creating a cyclical feedback loop, sending signals to the orbital frontal cortex that, in turn, registers a sense of dread that something is horribly wrong. The caudate nucleus also sends signals to the anterior cingulate gyrus that is connected to parts of the brain that control the heart and the stomach. This creates a physiological response of gut-churning, heart-racing anxiety that is reinforced again by the sense of dread registered in the orbital frontal cortex. Health comes when the gate is opened again for the normal flow of information. For OCD patients, the gate is difficult to reopen. One can become trapped in obsessive, unreasonable, ritualistic worrying (see chapter 3 for the SHIFT ritual designed specifically for OCD.)

Building a Treatment Program for Fear

Sometimes, reality teaches that our fears are well founded. Probably the most helpful emotional path out of fear begins with fatigue/rest/sleep or calming down from fear. Both anger and fear reduce our mind's working parts to the small mammalian brain. Relaxing helps us begin to incorporate our frontal lobe and aids our ability to think as well as feel. Teaching clients the skill of self-soothing is perhaps the most important tool we can give them to help them with fear.

Clients who have the best chance of becoming well-adjusted adults are those who manage their fears and anxieties in a healthy way with self-soothing skills. We can play an essential role in helping clients develop these skills, which are

- the ability to frame fears;
- the ability to undo negative predictions;
- the ability to use the imagination to focus away from the fear;
- the ability to use rituals for physical and emotional relaxation.

These self-soothing skills will provide a lifetime of emotional resources to our clients.

Framing Fears

Fearful personalities can be inherited. We can help clients put their fearful natures into the context of their families. Obsessive worry also can be an inherited trait. We should ask our worrying clients if their parents, grandparents, aunts, and uncles were worriers. Odds are you will find someone they know and love who fits this pattern. Clients don't feel so strange when they know that others before them have coped and thrived in spite of this shared problem with fearfulness or worry.

Undoing Negative Predictions

After we have framed our clients' fearfulness (fears named and associated with family heritage), focus on their negative predictions. Here, we must do battle with our clients' negative predictions by posing positive possible future outcomes as well. Remember, many negative predictions are reasonable. Driving 100 mph could be fatal. This negative prediction makes sense. Examine negative predictions. Ask the client who is afraid of airplanes what happened to the last person he knew who flew in a plane?

With questions such as these and using Yvonne Agazarian's fork-in-the-road technique, described earlier, we give our clients competing visions of the future. And we help them remember that they cannot predict or know the future. With "not knowing" in place of catastrophizing, we can encourage clients to ask the question of surprise, wonder, and mystery that will engage their curiosity. While surprised and curious, clients can avoid negative predictions and proceed to test fate and to discover what the future holds.

Make Fear the Teacher

There are two kinds of courage: fool's courage and informed courage. Taking a risk simply to prove to ourselves and others that we are not afraid is a form of fool's courage. Instead, we should help clients use fear to create an intelligent plan of action.

Fear is often a jumping-off place for panic. But fear also can become a Socratic teacher—one who teaches by asking questions. And asking questions is a means of putting fear in the proper perspective, reducing panic and soothing the self.

Asking questions and modeling curiosity can help clients see that fear does not close off options; rather, fear is the place to begin to ask questions: "What am I really afraid of? What do I know about the thing I fear? How can I find out more about the object of my fear?" With the expression of questions like these, fear becomes a starting point from which to gather information to support the courage they will need to move toward the object of their fear.

If your clients are afraid of snakes, help them learn about snakes. Ask them to find out which snakes are dangerous. Can they tell the poisonous ones from harmless, even helpful snakes? Refer them to the library or the Internet to learn about snakes and encourage them to discover ways of distinguishing which snakes are dangerous. As they learn about snakes, help them begin to develop a plan to face their fear of snakes. This would involve some form of systematic desensitization, associating the object of their fear, in this instance snakes, with relaxation.

The next step is to help clients build a plan of action for facing their fears and then going after their personal goals. Don't reassure them that the negative outcome of their fears won't happen. You can, however, help them think through their fears, using their fears to make a sensible plan to move forward. Their fears can provide the structure of a plan. Fears point out the obstacles that they must overcome to succeed, and the plan must offer ways to remove these obstacles.

Sometimes fear creates so much mental static that problems once easily solved by your clients are now beyond them when gripped with fear. Normally, therapists should avoid problem-solving and advice. But with fearful clients who have not yet developed self-soothing skills, we need to carefully offer our good sense and problem-solving skills.

Avoid becoming invested in your clients' accountability. Therapists do not need to assume the role of judge or parent. If clients don't follow through on the plan, it is because the plan does not create small enough, doable steps. It is not the clients' fault. It is the plan's fault—your fault for expecting too much as you helped them develop their plan.

Be patient. Fall back. Rethink the plan. Take the ego blow yourself. Create a new plan with a smaller next step that your clients believe they can manage.

Make Imagination the Safety Zone: Feelings—Image—Words

Sometimes we see children who are afraid for what seems to us no reason. Often night and sleep frighten children. Even though they are exhausted, they are afraid to go to sleep. For children, there is only a fine line between sleep and death. Faced with an exhausted and irritable child who refuses to go to sleep, we should be patient. Remember that getting through the night alone sometimes can be difficult for adults as well.

Imagination most often fuels fears. It brings back memories of danger. It creates all kinds of ideas of wrong things that can happen. It is important to shut down this engine of fear and to transform imaginations into a useful resource for calming fears and to help clients use their imaginations to create new, hopeful possibilities of future options.

Alternatively, we can encourage clients to use their imaginations as a way to distract them from their fears. This is the dissociation defense. It helps them detach from their fears. We can also help them use their imaginations to express their feelings. Bottled-up fears simply create more fears. We can guide clients in using their imaginations to transform fears into something outside their minds, something separate from themselves that they can fight rather than something inside that they can't comprehend or face.

Ask your clients to imagine that their fear is a monster or a demon. Tell them to describe it, name it, draw it, tell a story about it. In their story, ask them to create an ending in which they overcome their monster or demon. For example, clients can imagine that their fear is a leopard and that they are a powerful lion that can defeat a leopard. Or, as you ask them to imagine their fear and they imagine their fear to look like a leopard, they might then imagine their leopard actually is a monkey in disguise.

Some clients have a strong religious faith. Encourage them to use their faith to soothe their fears. Pray with them if you can. Suggest that they read their holy books to help them find calm. For Christians and Jews, the Twenty-third Psalm can be a useful passage.

Help your clients discover a transitional object that can calm them. One of my colleagues, Peter Scanlan, gives clients a rock and asks them to carry it with them. When they become frightened, he tells them to rub the rock with their thumb and forefinger and think of him being with them. They can feel the rock and talk with him, and, in their imagination, they will hear his voice talking to them, calming them.

Instead of allowing fears to run wild in our clients' imaginations, encourage them to use these tools to direct their imaginations and contain their fears.

Relaxation Techniques

All therapists are familiar with the relaxation response, a technique borrowed from the tradition of hypnosis. It distracts us from our fears and helps us relax. Often, there is little we can do about our fears. Focusing on them only makes matters worse. Teaching your clients the relaxation response will help them begin to sleep or at least to relax and remove some of the tension from their bodies.

There are many sources that teach the relaxation response, including *The Relaxation Response* by Herbert Benson (1975). But several other techniques create the same beneficial alpha brain waves (Bernstein & Borkovec, 1973). Basically, they all follow the same procedure but bear different names, such as chanting, meditation, self-hypnosis, and the name that sounds the most scientific, the relaxation response.

These methods have three things in common. One is diaphragmatic breathing or breathing naturally deep in the lungs. The second is a focus on the body, limb by limb, body segment by body segment (for example: relax toes, feet, ankles, calves, thighs, buttocks, lower back, mid-back, upper back, shoulders, fingers, hands, forearms, upper arms, neck, back of the head, top of the head, temples, jaw muscles, forehead, mouth).

The third is an emptying of the mind of thoughts (fears) or wants that create tension. Biofeedback focuses the mind on machines, teaching the client how to use the machines and this relaxed body state to control, for example, heart rate, galvanic skin response, muscle tension, and so forth. Meditation uses a mantra or chanting to empty the mind of all thought. Hypnosis uses a voice from a tape recorder, often the voice of a therapist. Once clients have begun diaphragmatic breathing, ask them to remember in their imaginations a time and a place when they felt relaxed and safe. Ask them to pretend that they are there and to stay there for 20 minutes in their mind—protected, loved, and relaxed. There is now a computer game called *The Journey to Wild Divine* that teaches relaxation with biofeedback.

By now, as a therapist, you probably have developed your own relaxation routine to use with clients. That routine is fine. The objective is to enable your clients to build this skill for themselves. They need to practice their own relaxation routine until they are competent at calming themselves with this tool. Of course, once this is in their own psychological toolboxes, with the therapist's guidance, they can incorporate it in managing phobias and obsessions.

Physical Relaxation Tools

Movement   Almost any physical energy release will vent our anxious energy. We will consider two major forms of exercise for reducing anxiety.

The first of these is aerobic exercise. Aerobic exercise builds heart rate, increases breathing, and releases endorphins. It also distracts us from our fears for a moment, puts us back in our human bodies, and renders the illusion of our being God (that is to say, able to control life) nearly impossible. The effect of the release of endorphins is a decreased number of worried and painful thoughts and increased feelings of euphoria and well-being. Endorphins are chemically closely related to morphine and other narcotics—yet they originate inside the brain.

Proponents of Eye Movement Desensitization Reprocessing (EMDR) suggest that rhythmical aerobic exercise, alternating from the right to the left side, has the effect of rapid eye movement (REM) that occurs in the alpha state of sleep. No one is sure how this happens, but speculation has it that REM and perhaps rhythmical exercise, such as walking or running, helps the brain process trauma.

The second form of exercise that releases stress is stretching. When the major muscle masses of the body are stretched, another natural narcotic called serotonin, as well as endorphin B, is released in the body. These biofluids relax our muscles and calm our bodies. Stretching also releases lactic acid and other toxins and renews muscles, preparing them to work with flexibility as well as strength.

When we are anxious, we can take advantage of this natural phenomenon. When we stretch, our muscles relax automatically, and we relax as well. Stretching has many real-life parallels. When we stretch, we put our bodies at risk. But if we stretch slowly to the edge of our pain, our muscles begin to expand, and we expand the limits of what we can do and how far we can reach.

As we focus internally on pushing our bodies' limits, we are controlling ourselves and our bodies. When we stretch, we are so absorbed in this discipline that we cannot focus on controlling others or life events. We must detach from our emotions and thoughts as we stretch .We must focus on our body and the fine line between the painful stretching sensation and hurt that is part of real injury. Stretching requires that we attend to the sensation in our bodies in the present moment.

The Dead-Face Trick

If you cannot find a place to stretch or time to walk, there is another way to relax the body that actors call the "dead-face trick." This "trick" takes away the remains of the previous emotions and prepares the actor for his next emotional acting challenge. It functions much as sorbet does to cleanse the palate between the courses of a gourmet meal. In the same way, the dead-face trick can relax our bodies, releasing our emotions.

Ekman (1977), Izard (1971), and Tomkins (1962) have demonstrated that the facial muscles have special neurological circuits that are connected to the brain. They hypothesized that our face registers our emotions first, and our brain reacts to the expression of the muscles in our face. Whether or not that is true, clearly the face has a central part to play in our emotional lives.

Consequently, if we want to feel relaxed, we can relax our face, and, in turn, we will relax. Here is the procedure for the dead-face trick:

> Sit down, close your eyes, and place your nondominant hand (left or right) at the top of your forehead. Bring your hand slowly and lightly down, across the surface of your face. As you bring your hand down from your forehead to your chin, allow your facial muscles to relax, making your face emotionless. For 20 or 30 seconds, keep your eyes closed and experience the sensation of a relaxed, expressionless face. Your body's sensation will follow the emotional instructions of the facial muscles, and your body will relax as your face does.

Friends, Family, and Pets

Among the tools clients can use to fight fear are friends, family, and pets. The research on stress clearly indicates the importance of social networks to our health, in part because sharing with friends our feelings of fear protects our health (Thoits, 1983). Affective bonds stimulate the cingulate cortex, which has a high concentration of opiate receptors. "Strong attachments increase endogenous opiates" (Buck, 1999, p. 35), thus helping us to relax.

In the spring of 2000, one of ABC-TV's *20/20* segments highlighted the use of helper dogs for people who suffer from social phobias. Clearly, such pets create attachment bonds. Also, the dogs that work with clients distract them from their fears and give them a sense of power and control, at least over the adoring dog. My dog Greco gives me this feeling of love and confidence, for which I am grateful.

Resolving Fear

By now, you should be wondering about emotional paths that can resolve fear. *Anger* is a great resource. It is the other half of fight/flight in the brain. Anger brings confidence and poise rather than the doubt and confusion of fear. The problem with anger is that frightened people can rarely access it. *Shame* is often a consequence of fear. Shame and fear together can form a dangerous pathological emotional knot. Shame, therefore, is a poor choice for resolving fear. Sadness, when connected to fear, also can create more problems and is not a good resource for resolving fear. *Sadness* and fear can oscillate back and forth, exhausting our minds and hearts, depleting us of norepinephrine (NE), and increasing the corticotropin releasing factor (CRF), thus locking us in chronic depression and obsessive fears (Risch, 1991).

If anger is not available, if shame and sadness only increase the brain's pain and pathology around fear, then what's left?

Surprise might work, but only to distract us. Surprise can sometimes increase the body's tension and magnify fears.

Interest/excitement? What about that emotion? Yes, that one is better, but fear usually blocks us from getting what we want. And caring and wanting can increase pressure and magnify fear.

Disgust? You can be afraid and feel disgust. But you had better not let the person you are afraid of see your disgust, or you risk precipitating an attack. Disgust implies a position of strength. Often when we are afraid, we do not have the strength to access disgust.

Joy, sure. But how easy is it to get from fear to joy without calming the fears in some way? Remember why rape doesn't satisfy a desire of the victim? That's because fear at high levels is incompatible with interest and joy. You must be somewhat calm and relaxed to feel pleasure.

This leads us to *fatigue/sleep/relaxation*. Yes, this is the best first step in creating new body hormones and transforming a tense body into a calm, relaxed body. This will bring the oxytocin, serotonin, and GABA that are associated with rest and the activation-parasympathetic activity.

The CALMS Ritual

I was so impressed by the clarity and simplicity of Stosny's HEALS technique that I used a similar acronym to treat fear. I call it the CALMS meditation. It includes the following steps:

1. Stop the catastrophizing and induce the not-knowing, surprise/wonder state in which dangerous predictions are balanced by positive possibilities.
2. Use fear to create a plan to go toward interest/excitement.
3. Loosen the body and prepare it to relax.
4. Introduce the relaxation response. Meditate.
5. Move toward what we want, use the plan made in Step 2, and follow that plan.

Following is the CALMS meditation that I describe in the CALMS manual, which I developed for use in my practice.

Step 1: Confess. To begin, we must confess that we are not God. We can't control destiny. We don't know the future. We don't know the outcomes of our efforts. Positive outcomes might be available to us in the future, as well as negative ones. Return from the future to the fork-in-the-road of the present and be curious. Make the unknown the neutral place that it is.

 Step 2: Approach. Approach your fears with curiosity. Learn about the object of your fears. As you move toward a fear, obstacles will emerge. These obstacles are things we must overcome to succeed. Design a plan to deal with these obstacles. The plan should include several small, doable steps. Be sure that the first step is small enough for you to begin the approach without being overcome by fear.

 Step 3: Loosen the body. This requires exercise. Emphasize stretching the large muscle groups. Aerobic exercise also helps prepare us to relax. For many of us, time is short. Sometimes when we need to calm ourselves, we don't have a place or time to exercise. It's important to do what we can to relax our bodies. Stretching is an excellent choice.

 Step 4: Meditate. Our minds are prepared, and our bodies are relaxed. Begin relaxed, diaphragmatic breathing. Now we are ready to meditate. Here, for 5 minutes, we exchange anxious thoughts for our mantra. Mantra is a phrase or sound that we repeat over and over slowly that blocks all thoughts. This exchange of thoughts for mantra defeats fear with faith. Every time a fear thought enters our mind and does not create tension in the body, we defeat fear and replace it with a neutral thought—the mantra—giving us the internal message: For now, we are safe.

 Step 5: Start something. Follow the plan of approach. Move toward your goal. Take action, even a small step to get started. Do something to address your concerns and go after what you want, using your fears to create a plan instead of being confined by them.

These treatment notions are not revolutionary. Most therapists suggest these actions when they help clients with fears and phobias. The contribution of this chapter is that it provides a theoretical way of understanding why what we therapists have always done works. It also gives us a clear understanding of why, heuristically, relaxation must be part of any treatment taxonomy of emotions. Without relaxation, we cannot effectively treat fear.

Summary and Conclusion

I saw Anthony for some 7 months. At our last session Anthony said, "I've learned a lot here, Dr. McMillan. But of all the things that I learned, the CALMS technique was the best. I can now relax, on my own, by myself, no pills, I can put myself in a trance and turn down my anxiety. And that's a great thing. And now, I can fly on an airplane. That was a good thing we did, going to the airport and practicing the CALMS technique inside a plane, with the engine on, then taxiing down the runway without taking off. And then, when we took off, I didn't know it! We were in the air, and I was relaxed, and then I looked out the window, and I had to do the CALMS technique for 15 minutes before I calmed down, but I did.

"I got a dog. That was your suggestion. Bud, my dog, really helped me meet people and be comfortable. The focus is on the dog, and I can talk about Bud forever. Bud's so smart and can do such mischief. Anyway, I can fly, meet clients, but girls still scare me. Do you think I'll get over that?"

"I don't know," I said, "but the opposite sex scares most of us. It just means that women are really important to you. That's not a bad thing. Keep focusing on controlling your fears and calming yourself, and I think you will even find a woman you can trust."

CHAPTER 7

Sadness
The Most Paralyzing Emotion

Sadness Defined

Sadness is a response to loss and separation from what we desire and need. Our body has certain constant states that make up our physical and emotional equilibrium. When we lose the essentials of our physical and emotional constants, we are sad (Tomkins, 1962). Losing food, shelter, and clothes creates sadness, as does losing what we love. Sadness is the central emotion in the grief process (Izard, 1971). Sadness attracts comfort. Parents of a crying infant want to offer nurture and comfort (Greenberg & Paivio, 1997). The tears of our friends cause us to open our arms to them. As they feel sad, we feel sad with them. Sadness reflects how much we care about what we lost (Nathanson, 1992). The greater we care, the greater our sadness. Sadness cleanses, renews, and reconnects us with love (Greenberg, 2001).

Sadness is a recognition that we can't have what we want. It tells us to "let go," "give it up," "accept the fact that. . . ," "you'll have to start over." It is what we do after a loss before we refocus our energy on a new goal and a different desire. It is the process we go through to put the past in its place. Though painful, sadness can teach us what we need to know to be successful in our next venture.

Clinical Case Study

I first saw Kay when she was a high school student. Recently she returned to see me because her mother had committed suicide and she wanted help. Now she was 30 years old with a daughter of her own, 6-year-old Terri.

"I'm sad, but I'm beyond sad," Kay said. "I'm angry. I'm afraid. I am lost. She was my constant. She was my rock. How could she want to die? I could never leave Terri on purpose. Was I not enough? Yes, I feel guilty, too. My mental balance, what there is of it, was given to me by her love I took it for granted. It was always a steady stream.

"Even her suicide was kind. While my father was out of town, she left a note for the cleaning lady and one for me and my dad. In the note for the cleaning lady, she told her to call the police and tell them that she had checked into the Holiday Inn and had taken an overdose of pills; by the time she read this note, Mother wrote, she would be dead.

"In the note to me, she told me how proud of me she was, what a good mother I had become, what a good wife I was, what a fine career I had built, that I didn't really need her now, and she couldn't fight this depression anymore. She had to go. "Please forgive me," she asked.

"Well, I don't. She can't decide that I don't need her. That's for me to say. She has always been proud of me, whether I was playing volleyball or losing an election for vice president of my class. Now, I can't count on her to be proud of me even in my next failure.

"I won't forgive her. I won't get over this. I don't want to feel good. I expect to feel sad the rest of my life. I don't want to fill this hole in my heart. I treasure this hole. Now it is all I have left of her. I will never stop missing her. I will always be sad.

"But it's been 18 months since she died, and I cry about her every day. I've got to get over this; my husband is tired of it. My daughter needs a happy mother. I'm afraid I've got my mother's depression. I don't want to take any pills."

Neurology of Sadness

Sadness in the brain is often treated by researchers as the negative end of the polarity of happy/sad. It is focused in the limbic system, especially in the septal thalamocingulate, the anterior hypothalamus, the ventromedial hypothalamus (VM), and the medial forebrain bundle (MFB) (Maas, 1975). Sadness is associated with greater right frontal activity and diminished level of activity in the left frontal portion of the brain. Sadness tends to increase lateralization in the brain through the lateral ventricular, thus incorporating both sides of the brain in the experience of this emotion (Steingard, et al., 1996). The right hemisphere searches for changes in the environment. It alerts the brain to novelty. This is in contrast to the left hemisphere that is biased toward noticing patterns, trends, and redundancies (Tucker & Williamson, 1984). Since the right hemisphere is more active during sadness, the brain appears to be searching for something new that will pull us out of sadness and into interest and hope.

Low levels of norepinephrine (NA), serotonin (5-H7), oxytocin (OXY), and dopamine (DA) are associated with sadness. High levels of corticotrophin-releasing factor (CRF), peptide neurotransmitters, monoamine oxidase (MAO), and substance P (the carrier of the pain message) are associated with sadness (Redmond & Murphy, 1975). The brain treats loss and physical pain similarly. In fact, pain is the signal of the loss of a steady state in the body.

Physiology of Sadness

The function of sadness is to slow the cognitive and motor systems so that we can have "a more careful look for the source of trouble, (reflect deeper) or a disappointing performance or failure" (Izard & Ackerman, 1999, p. 258). Sadness slows breathing and heart rate, lowers blood pressure, and raises finger temperature. Skin-conductance level improves, and the body falls asleep more easily.

The face drops to express sadness. The upper lip might quiver. The mouth droops. Tears are markers of sadness; the sensation that one is about to cry is also a characteristic sadness response. Sometimes, the nose will wrinkle, the head will drop, and eyes will focus downward.

The Negative Consequences of Sadness

Sadness is so neurologically connected to pain that it is difficult to find ways to express its negative consequences other than to say that it hurts. There are a great many philosophical platitudes about sadness and wisdom, and they are all true. But the bottom line is that it hurts.

Chronic sadness, like chronic back pain, colors our perception of the world. Things look dark. Hope becomes a rare commodity. Interest and libido, sexual or otherwise, fade. It is hard to believe that we can be successful at anything. When we are sad, often the best we can do is emerge from despair into cynicism.

Sadness is associated with the cancer personality (Easterling & Leventhal, 1989). (Other correlates of the cancer personality are denial of anger and a tendency to put the needs of others first.) In health problems, we see sadness at work when one part of a couple, who have been married for 50 years, dies and their life partner dies within a week. Poor medical compliance is also a by-product of sadness, for example, heart attack clients who won't stop smoking (Glaus & Schwartzman, 2000).

Sadness often is concurrent with low self-esteem and self-hatred. It is the major emotion in depression. Sadness is associated with irritability in an agitated depression.

When people repeatedly play their sadness card in social situations, they drive away their friends. Friends want to bring comfort to their sad friends, but only if they can see that the comfort that they bring matters. If it doesn't, they will go away.

The Positive Consequences of Sadness

Sadness is the soap of our emotional system. Its tears and the comfort that sadness attracts can wash away the poison of anger, fear, and shame.

When we are sad, we have at least begun the process of letting go of something we wanted but couldn't have. We are no longer afraid of losing it, because we know that it is indeed lost. We are no longer angrily fighting for it, because we recognize fighting is useless. We are sometimes sad, because in our shame we have lost our dignity. Our tears help us acknowledge wrongdoing and begin the process of rebuilding trust.

Facing loss is a difficult emotional task. Most people experience several emotional stages in the work we call "grief." At first, we might vent our anguish through tears, an experience that can be exhausting for anyone who has suffered serious losses.

When we weep, we are communicating our distress and anguish to others. That is why the expression "a good cry" often is used. It describes weeping that brings comfort and help from others. It is also the reason why weeping sometimes creates discomfort in other people. When we don't know how to offer help to someone who is crying, or when we don't want to, for one reason or another, their tears burden us precisely because their tears are a request for help that we do not know how to give.

When we want to avoid asking others for help, we often seek privacy to weep, a place where we can hide the tears that might guilt-induce sympathy that we don't want. To understand the power of tears in bringing help, just think of a crying baby. Infants have no other means of getting help except by crying for it, and usually their tears prove highly effective.

Sadness honors the thing, person, or outcome that we have lost. For example, if your mother died and if you are proud that you loved your deceased mother deeply, you will not be ashamed of your tears. Your sadness simply reflects the depth of your love. In this context, you are proud to show how much your mother meant to you and how much you will miss her.

Sadness and Intelligence

There are conflicting opinions on whether sadness promotes intelligence. Clearly sadness helps a formerly angry brain cleanse itself of the good/bad, black/white, two-category thinking of anger. Sadness helps us resolve anger and see reality more clearly (Stosny, 1995; Schneider, 1956). Others note research on depressed clients that documents decrease in I.Q. when depressed (Cicchetti & Toth, 1998). Sadness is marked by decreased activity in the prefrontal cortices (Damasio, 1994).

I would suggest that the decrease in I.Q. that is associated with depression is a reflection of the famous bell-curve relationship between anxiety and performance. Depressed clients in mental hospitals often do not care enough to attend or to perform well on intelligence tests. Persons who are merely sad (not in a clinical depression) have a greater access to their brain and their best common sense, as they reflect on reality in the context of their sadness.

Sadness relaxes us, while it sensitizes us to reality. The sadness neurostructure does not include the amygdala, which seems either to confuse us or give us false confidence. Sad circuitry goes from the brainstem to the neocortex. Sadness touches every level of the brain, calming us by taking away the static that can come from fear and anger. In sadness, we have access to all of the brain's I.Q. if we want to use it, but generally we don't.

Sadness and Grief

Reading Elisabeth Kübler-Ross's *On Death and Dying* (1969) and her description of the five stages of grief was another moment of insight for me in understanding how emotions move from one to another in a process of healing. The five stages of grief are denial, bargaining, anger, sadness, and acceptance. Of course, these are not pure stages that move precisely from one to another. One can go from anger to denial or from acceptance to bargaining. But generally Kübler-Ross described well the flow of emotions during the grief process.

In *denial*, the pain of reality is too much to absorb, so we pretend it isn't so. I remember when my beloved eldest brother, Bill, died in a car accident along with his girlfriend. I was 14 years old. Shortly after their deaths, I was walking alone on the golf course late in the day, approaching my ball on the fairway. I told myself as I walked that it wasn't true, that this was just a dream, and that even as I was walking toward my ball that I was dreaming I was playing golf. I was not playing golf. I was really asleep, and my brother Bill was alive.

I decided to put my bag down and pinch my butt as hard as I could. If I felt pain, I was awake. If later a bruise appeared, it would mean that Bill was really dead. I pinched myself. It hurt, and I got a bruise. Today I still don't want to believe it.

Consider this example. A woman discovers that her husband is having an affair but denies that his infidelity troubles her. She might tell herself, "It makes no difference. He's still a good provider," or, "He's still a good father," or, "That other woman means nothing to him," or "He's not having an affair. They are just good friends." She denies the significance of the facts that stare her in the face in order to protect herself against the hurt of the important loss of trust.

Children, as well, often use denial as a defense. It is common, for instance, for a child to say, "I don't care, whatever," when questioned about a situation that has probably created sadness. Children might feign indifference when a parent returns after a long trip, or deny that it matters to them when a parent is late, forgets an important date, or cannot participate in a school activity because of work. Usually, the indifferent "I don't care" signals parents that their child is denying the feeling of loss, that he or she does want something and is disappointed not to get it.

Denial often works for a while to protect us from sadness. But it is hard work to keep denial in place. The true feelings of loss continue popping up unexpectedly, often when our defenses are down. And, also, our friends usually don't buy it. They ask questions that arouse our feelings of loss. No matter how often we deny these feelings, reality does not go away.

The second stage of grief is *bargaining*. In that stage we believe that we lost one round of the fight but did not lose the cause. With more sacrifice and a better attitude, the victory still could be ours. Classically, bargaining manifests itself in what some call "foxhole religion." People pray in a crisis. Their prayer is an attempt to bargain with God. If God will make reality be different than it is, then we will...for God. Danny Thomas, a famous TV entertainer from the 1960s, made such a prayer once and the creation of St. Jude Hospital in Memphis was the result of his keeping his promise. Most of the time bargaining doesn't change reality.

The next stage is a *temper tantrum*. We become angry at God, angry at the person who died, angry at the person who accidentally ran into our car. And we remain angry, until we see that the energy our anger brings us is not changing the facts we must face.

Once we see that, we can't deny reality, we cannot bargain our way into a different reality, and we cannot fight fate with anger. At this point, we are resigned to *feeling the sadness*, processing the pain, learning from our experience, and moving to the next step—which is *acceptance*, acceptance that we lost and must begin again, working within the confines of what we now know to be true.

Probably most therapists know this grief recipe by heart. What it taught me is how healthy and natural is the connection between anger and sadness. It is obvious, once you understand the grief process, that anger protects us from sadness and that sadness naturally follows anger.

Neurologically this is true. Think about how we feel after we have been in a fit of anger. Sad is how most of us would respond, because anger quickly depletes us of adrenaline and noradrenaline. Sadness is what we naturally feel when these autonomic nervous system chemicals are low in the body (Roth, 1994). And this makes sense, too, because sadness slows down the body and promotes rest, giving the body a chance to replenish itself after an angry burst of energy.

Surviving Loss

In the last stage of healthy grief, we retrace our previous defenses. Once again, as when we cried, we hold fast to sadness and the feeling of loss, but now we do so in order to affirm that what we lost was important. As when we raged, we feel angry that something so valuable was lost, but now we use our anger as determination to find a new way to succeed.

We call on our imagination to envision a way to use the wisdom gained from our pain. We explore how to survive our loss in a way that allows us to risk wanting again. We begin to see how to add new hope to our sadness, hope that was once denied. With our determination and what we have learned from our loss, our new hope has a chance of being realized.

Clearly, grief is a complicated process, and our clients often require help in identifying and experiencing the various strands of feelings that are involved in this process.

Resolving Sadness

Joy is on the other end of the neurological polarity with sadness (Buck, 1999). Certainly, joy can resolve sadness. But for this to happen we must snatch victory from the jaws of defeat or raise Lazarus from the dead. Usually that is not possible. Joy is an excellent destination, but often it is not a realistic next move from sadness.

Disgust is an evaluative emotion that finds good in some things and rejects others. It is intellect more than energy, which makes it difficult to reach disgust from sadness. If disgust is combined with anger and we can be in a strong position, disgust can become a part of the path that resolves sadness. But combined with anger, disgust can make us act impulsively and can cast us to shame. Rarely can we move in a healthy way from sadness to the strong position disgust might provide.

Shame and *sadness* cover much of the same neurological territory. They both hurt. Their function is to stop us or slow us down. Shame offers no energy. Shame and sadness together create a deep emotional hole. It is a poor choice as a next step out of sadness.

Fatigue/rest as emotion is the opposite of arousal and awake. Sleep can renew the body, but not the soul. Sad people often try to play Rip van Winkle and sleep long enough so that when they awake, their problems will be gone. Unfortunately, few of us can successfully sleep our troubles away. Using sleep to avoid pain most often lengthens the amount of time we are sad.

Sadness is an emotional place that is devoid of energy. It is a place where effort will not work. We accept that there is nothing we can do. Hence, to get out of sadness, we must find a source of energy.

Four emotions give us energy. One is *fear*. Fear may help us resolve sadness if we can use our fear to help us develop a plan of action that will yield success and joy. But too often fear paralyzes us rather than provides us direction. Fear can create energy that has nowhere to go. Sadness will at least allow us to rest. It is difficult for us to rest when we are also afraid. Fear is usually a poor choice.

The second emotion that provides us energy is *interest/excitement/desire*. Sadness is boring. Usually we tire of sadness after a time. We want to refocus our attention from what made us sad to something we want (interest/excitement/desire). But often we are discouraged, and we have no faith that we actually can have anything we want.

Wanting is a good next step out of sadness, if we have the courage to want again after losing what we once desired but could not have. To want again, we must find a new, reasonably achievable desire. The object of our desire is irrelevant. We need to find something that we want that will lift us out of our depression stupor.

The third emotion that can create energy is *anger*. Anger is a most effective next step out of sadness. Many of us naturally gravitate to anger when we are sad. Men are socialized to use anger to avoid sadness so that they never cry. Remember, "real men don't cry." But what they can do is have a temper tantrum like a 5-year-old.

Anger has the energy, confidence, and focus that we need to emerge from sadness and back into life. Anger alone can be stupid and lead us to shame and hence back to sadness. If, however, we hold on to the wisdom of sadness and remember that our anger is stupid, we can play with our anger, turning the circumstances into a fantasy cartoon in our minds. This form of imaginary play can become an excellent energy source.

Surprise is also an emotion that creates energy. But we cannot create a surprise. By definition, if we are in control and expect something to happen, that something will not surprise us. Even if we are startled out of depression, surprise likely will merge with fear, which probably will not resolve sadness. Or, surprise will be quickly resolved, and we will return to sadness.

To help us out of sadness, we should use a combination of three emotions interest/excitement/desire, anger, and joy. Joy, of course, is the destination. In the ritual suggested here, interest initiates our arousal and anger potentates the power of our arousal. This combination in a different order is familiar to most of us at the end of a romantic relationship. Sadness results from the romantic breakup. Anger provides the healing protection of a scab to a wound. When interest in someone or some new activity emerges, often the anger disappears and we can establish a new, healthy emotion flow. In this process, we should not completely forget our sadness. Sadness brings us the gift of wisdom and good sense. We should retain what our sadness taught us. Our sadness can leaven our anger so that we do not take our anger seriously but only use our anger as part of a playful fantasy.

These emotions—interest/excitement/desire, anger, and sadness—are the ingredients of determination. Determination contains the wisdom of sadness, the energy of anger, and the sense of direction from interest. It may also include courage, which is a combination of fear, anger, and desire. Determination will keep us moving forward, picking us up when we fall. With determination, we will eventually reach joy and resolve sadness.

The ALIVE Ritual

Psychologists discovered this combination of emotions, though they never discussed it as I do here. Freud saw depression as the absence of libido or what I call interest/excitement/desire. On this Freud and I agree. The treatment he taught his disciples was to be present for the patient, sit with her several times a week without saying much. In this quiet, the patient discovers a personal agenda. They become so frustrated with the lack of interaction with the therapist who was supposed to help them that they get angry. They become their own authority and terminate their treatment determined (anger + desire) to live their own lives as they see fit.

I agree with this analytic treatment goal. I think, however, we can tell our clients how emotions work, and they often can come up with solutions of their own.

I developed another five-step acronym for treating excessive sadness and clinical depression. For people who are trapped in a depression cycle and are ready to try a new approach, the ALIVE ritual works well. But for people for whom depression creates secondary gain, it doesn't work (secondary gains are benefits that are gained secondarily from the symptom). Beyond this, certain individuals have a fearful, depressed personality style and refuse to use anger in any way. Such individuals cannot use the ALIVE ritual, because it requires them to engage their anger.

Before we recommend this methodology, we should remember three things:

1. Some sadness is healthy. It can be tender and sweet, teach us wisdom, and bring compassion to us from others.

2. Many individuals who recruit sadness as their primary emotion cannot use anger in any form. The following procedure will be difficult for them to use.

3. Anger is stupid. When clients engage anger, they should not take their anger seriously. They should imagine that they are drawing a cartoon in their minds, creating caricatures. It is an imaginary play exercise. If your clients cannot understand the use of imaginary play as a fantasy exercise, do not use the ALIVE ritual.

Following is The Alive ritual[8] that I have developed for my clients:

 Step 1: **A**wareness of something that you want. If you are having trouble knowing what you want, find a place to be alone. Sit in a comfortable chair. Relax and breathe. Place your attention on your ears, nose, mouth, and hands. Ask each of them what they want to sense: hear, smell, taste, or touch. Next, focus your attention on the center of your torso, either your solar plexus or your heart area, and ask your heart and soul what they want. Repeat this process until you have discovered something for which you long. Once you have identified what you want, go to Step 2. (If you are still having trouble locating a want, focus on your fears. Your fears give you the direction of your want. If you are afraid of flying, convert fear of flying into your want to fly. Continue to Step 2, using "I wish I could fly" as your want.) Find a simple and concrete want, something that can be achieved and is not abstract. (We are strongest when we are working on a goal that is within our boundaries. If our goal is to control someone else or to have a specific outcome from an event, we will likely fail since our only real opportunity for control is ourselves. Success or failure, however, is not as important as striving and learning.) Your task in this step of the process is to become turned on, awake, conscious, and alive: to want again, the simpler and more concrete a want the better.

Step 2: Learning from fear. Fear can easily push us back into sadness. It can also prepare and teach us. Make an action plan based on your fears. Focus on your fears. Learn from them what you need to know in order to prepare a good plan of attack for what you want to achieve. Prepare an action plan. Listen only to the fears that inform your plan and prepare you for action. Use logic and the perspective of others to test whether your fears are reasonable concerns or just excuses to remain stuck. Listen to reasonable concerns, as you build your campaign plan. Ignore the fears that are excuses. This step dismisses paralyzing fears and uses fear to help us have common sense.

 Step 3: Include faith in the process now. Change your negative core beliefs by discovering them. Are you unimportant? Of course, the answer is no. Worthy of disregard? No. Unlovable? No. Powerless? No. Build faith in yourself and your abilities. Tell the truth about yourself. Faith requires that we work to eliminate the habit of targeting ourselves with negative beliefs about our souls. There is truth in the bumper-sticker motto, "God didn't make junk." The basic ingredients of our souls are wholesome and wonderful. When we attack ourselves with painful statements about our character, we are lying. Your job is to be rigorously honest. Consider the core negative beliefs you have that you are: unimportant, unworthy, unlovable, powerless, inadequate and disgusting, or unfit for human contact. Once you have discovered your negative core belief, or beliefs, ask this question: Is it true that you are unimportant, unworthy, valueless, powerless or inadequate, unlovable, disgusting, or unfit for human contact? The answer is always, "No!"

Tell the truth and remind yourself of the reality of your existence and the value of your essential spirit to yourself and to the community. You may have made mistakes. Others might be angry and disappointed with you. They may even attempt to assassinate your character. But your character is your responsibility. You alone own your soul. You alone know your essential self. You alone can make judgments about your core self. Speak the truth of your importance, regard, worth, value, power, adequacy, lovability, and basic fitness for life. Speak aloud about your basic value. Then, write it down. Continue this until you realize your worth. This step protects you from toxic shame. Shame, if not challenged, can plunge you back into sadness and fear.

 Step 4: Vent your anger in fantasy, turning anger into determination to take care of yourself. Turn on anger. Look for an enemy,

someone who, as you imagine his or her face, makes your blood pressure rise. Target your anger at this villain, as if you were writing and drawing a comic book. You can be Batman, Xena, Spider-man, or Wonder Woman. In your fantasy, imagine lots of POW!s, BANG!s, WHOP!s, BLAM!s, and **&@#!!s**. This is play that turns on the most primitive parts of your brain. At first, this might appear to be a stupid exercise, but it sure is fun. As you proceed in your fantasy, look for the point at which you feel you have gone too far, even for a fantasy. When you get to this point, you have turned on the second part of your brain: the compassion/empathy adult part. Now, put your enemy back together in your fantasy. Talk to him or her. Watch for the place in the conversation where you say, "I don't really want to hurt you. I want you to stop hurting me, and I am determined to stay turned on and to fight for what I want and what I believe is right." When your imagination gets to this point, you have completed Step 4. You are turned on and ready for action. Do not engage your compassion before you get the energy you need from your anger.

 Step 5: <u>E</u>ngage yourself in action. Follow the plan you made in Step 2, the <u>L</u> step. That plan was informed by the wisdom of your fear. Jump in, get going. Do something. No excuses. Focus on the next step. You have a right to want and to go after your want. Be determined and strong.

Mothers Against Drunk Drivers (MADD) is an example of the ALIVE technique at work in a real situation. The founding members of this organization were grieving mothers whose children died because of drunk drivers. Their sadness was resolved by determined anger and a new interest—passing legislation that put people who drink and drive in jail. The founders of this organization visualized anger and revenge. They used the wisdom of their sadness to form an organization to prevent future pain for others, rather than pursuing personal revenge. This was a healthy emotional path out of sadness.

Sadness and Compassion

Carly Simon sings a song with the lyric: "There's more room in a broken heart."

Sadness does have something to do with love and our capacity for empathy. If I am a good therapist, it is not so much because of my training, though I am grateful for those who have guided and taught me this craft. My personal pain has been my main therapy teacher. When people come to me lost, sad, feeling alone, unable to stop the hurt, I can help them because I have felt that way, too.

Sadness deepens our ability to understand the pain of others. When we see others in psychic pain, we know better than to say, "Get over it." The experience of sadness tenderizes the soul and gives us wisdom. Part of the wisdom that sadness teaches is that to accomplish a goal we must understand how others feel. Sadness and loss force us to begin to look at reality from the perspective of others.

Many people are afraid of sadness and refuse to feel it when fate gives them the opportunity. They are the losers here. Sadness is an important part of growing up.

Life is a tragedy. We all pay taxes, and we all die. We need comfort from each other as we all face the pains of life: the surprises of fate, aging, and death. Sadness prepares us to be a kind, loving friend, parent, and mate. Sadness announces that we care.

Summary and Conclusion

I don't expect Kay will ever heal the hole in her heart left by her mother's death. I was sad for Kay, Terri, and Kay's mother, Terri's grandmother. But I did think Kay's depression had lasted far too long and was becoming dangerous. She needed to discover her other emotions, and she didn't know how.

"Try the ALIVE technique," I said, "It is just a ritual that will take about 5 minutes. Do it twice a day or more and let's continue working together for a while."

The next week she returned.

"I'm not comfortable with this ritual," she said. "I can't get angry. I'm like my mother that way."

"And that's why she couldn't get over her depression," I replied. "If you are sad and can't find the energy you get from anger, it is hard to move beyond depression."

"You mean my mother killed herself because she couldn't get angry. That's frightening."

"That's a bit too simple, I'm sure," I answered. "But often depressed people can only get angry at themselves. When that happens, there is no one to defend them against themselves. While if you got angry at me, for example, I could defend myself."

"Well, that gives me motivation to practice the ALIVE technique. If getting mad is something I need to learn, I need help. That ritual might work for me."

We met for several more weeks, and Kay practiced the ALIVE ritual. She became better at using it. On her last visit she said. "Boy, am I a bitch.

I jumped all over my husband last night for leaving his pants on the floor. Before, I wouldn't have said anything about that. I got on Terri's case about losing her new Game Boy. Before, I wouldn't have said anything much about that either.

"I'm not sure they like me better. But I'm taking dance lessons for the first time since I was 18—flamenco lessons. I love it. I thought that my husband would never allow this, but he seems unthreatened by my gay instructor.

"I think about my mother and how kind and supportive she was. I see now she was too kind. I wonder how many times she didn't get angry at me and my dad when she should have. I wonder how many times she abandoned her desires for ours. I wish she had practiced that ALIVE ritual. Though she might not have remained such a saint in my eyes, I think she would have still been here."

CHAPTER 8

Joy/Contentment
The Destination Emotion

Joy Defined

In considering joy, the emotion, we might confuse a sense of well-being, emotional balance, and personal fulfillment with happiness and joy. As we use these terms here, they do not mean the same thing. Remember, we are focusing on the emotion that we express through our face.

Joy is neither stupid nor dumb. It does not give specific action instructions; it prepares our brain to be at its best in playing, learning, or loving. Generally, joy relaxes and opens our mind so that it can function optimally.

Joy and happiness cover the same emotional territory. Joy is our destination emotion, and we all strive toward a goal that we believe will yield happiness. The joy that our faces reflect represents nine emotional experiences:

1. Joy of greeting, the smiles among strangers, meeting for the first time, indicating hope of friendship; the smiles of old friends, reunited.
2. Tears of joy, representing a victory requiring great sacrifices;
3. Predatory joy, merging the focus of desire with anger and eventually ending in the expression of joy at the victory of consumption;
4. Joy, witnessing the tragedy of another; our laughter, for example, when someone slips on a banana peel;
5. Joy of mastery upon learning a new skill;
6. Joy of creativity, when we invent something, design something, or make something that did not exist for us before;
7. Steady, mild joy or contentment; what we feel after the climactic, joyful celebration of a victory;

8. Joy of successful collaboration; the celebration of our achievements and those of friends, family, team, church, and country;

9. Communal joy, reflected in the welcoming smiles of friends reunited, of coming home, of the safety emanating from friends and loved ones coming together.

We humans cannot discern among these nine versions of joy simply by looking at another's face. Each of these sentiments is expressed with the same smile and laugh. Joy, therefore, is a word that represents them all.

Robert Provine's (2001) study of laughter documents the social function of joy. His primary point is that joy is not just the expression of genuine happiness. It is a face we put on that serves a social function. His study of laughter documents that speakers are 46% more likely to be laughing than are listeners. This implies that the purpose of the speaker's smiles and laughter is to influence the listener. Another part of Provine's study found that only 15% of laughter was stimulated by a funny event or statement. Most laughter, then, has a social function, communicating openness and a willingness to be friendly. Apparently we laugh and smile to encourage people to like us.

Children demonstrate that smiles are attractive. Their survival depends on their ability to create an attachment bond with an adult female with milk. Human infants begin to smile at about the time they are ready for solid food. The smile becomes the infants' vehicle for positive feedback. Notice the difference between the sounds of a group of children on a playground and the sounds of a grouping of adults. The difference is in the melody of laughter in the children. Laughter stimulates pleasure in the listener—laughter is contagious. "The largest amount of human laughter seems to occur in the midst of early childhood" (Pankseep, 2002; interview quoted by Johnson, 2004). A child's laughter is an important part of the parent/child glue that supports our young through their vulnerable developmental years.

Clinical Case Study

Virginia and Howard had been consulting me weekly, as a couple, for some 3 months. Therapy was about to reach a climax with this session.

"I don't seem to be able to get to Howard," Virginia began. "Nothing I do matters. I cook his favorite dessert. What does he say but, 'It's okay.' I ask him, 'How do you feel that I did this for you?' He says, 'Fine.' I ask him, 'Are you happy being married to me?' He answers, 'Sure, I'm always happy.' I could run off to Las Vegas with Howard's best friend, gamble away all our money, return, and Howard would still be happy."

"What's wrong with that?" Howard said. "I thought being happy was a good thing."

"See, he just doesn't get it. I want to matter to Howard. I want to make a difference. I want to contribute to his happiness, but how can you do that for somebody who is already happy? It's not only that he is happy. Howard knows everything. He never reads instructions or stops to ask for directions. Howard is master of his universe. Last year, we were on vacation and brought our digital camera. Howard hasn't used it much. He wants to change the setting. Did he ask me? No. Did he read the directions? No. Two weeks of pictures erased. All Maine erased, because Howard always knows what to do. Was he upset? No. Was I? Yes, and being upset made me a bitch. I feel like a bitch anytime I'm with Howard and I'm not happy. It's always, 'What's wrong with me? Why can't I be happy?'"

"Yes, that's right," Howard said. "We have a good home. I've got a good job. We have good friends. I'm tired of this. Nothing I ever do seems to make her happy. I've tried now for over 25 years, and I'm about ready to give up."

"What do you mean?" I asked.

"Well," Howard began, "we were living together. I was fine with that. But no, Virginia wanted to get married. She seemed so unhappy at the time, so I agreed. She was happy the day of the wedding, but 3 days later she was mad at the world and me. I married her, because I thought that marrying her would make her happy."

"Our dog died," Virginia blurted out. "Am I supposed to be happy when the Irish setter we had for 3 years dies? Howard would try to comfort me by saying, 'I love you.' I would try to ignore him, but he would just keep on saying it. 'Aren't you happy that I love you? Well, I do. I love you. I'm sorry our dog died, but I love you.'

"Howard's whole male ego rested on my responding to his 'I love you' with a smile, followed by, 'Yes, dear. It makes me very happy that you love me.' Our dog, Bo had just died, and Howard had to make me happy. I didn't want to be happy, and I didn't want to have to pretend to be happy, so that he would leave me alone and let me be sad. But that's what I did. I pretended that all that mattered was that he loved me, and I was happy because of that."

"Yeah, it's always something I do wrong. After the wedding, it was, 'I want to move to Nashville,'" Howard said. "She hated Dallas. 'Apply for that job at Vanderbilt. I will be closer to my family,' she said. I did. I got the job. But did that make her happy? No. Her mother was now too close and driving her crazy. So we had to move away from the university to Brentwood. That would be far enough from her mother. No matter that I had a 45-minute commute. She still wasn't happy.

"Then she wanted kids," Howard continued. "She said that would make her happy. We had two children, perfect children, a girl and a boy. The boy, George, has graduated from college and is getting his PhD in chemistry. Our girl, Cynthia, is in her senior year at Wake Forest. The children seemed to make her happy for a few years.

"But then she wanted a new house, an expensive home in Belle Meade. She had to have it. It was near where our children would be in school. No matter that I had to take on consulting work in addition to my work as a professor in the law school. Now do you know what she wants? She wants a new diamond, a three-carat, a $20,000 clear pebble. Will that make her happy? No. I'm tired. I give up," Howard concluded.

"It's our 25th wedding anniversary, Howard," Virginia countered. "I've borne you two children. Both our children went to college on full scholarship. We have the money. Why wouldn't you want to buy me a nice diamond now?"

"The reason I won't give you a diamond," responded Howard, "is that it won't make any difference. You will just want something else next week. I can't do anything that would make you happy."

Neurology of Joy

The poles of joy and sadness in the brain are in the medial forebrain (MFB) and the periventricular system (PVS) (LeGros, et al., 1938). As one is engaged, the other is turned off. Joy turns on the medial forebrain (MFB) and turns off the periventricular system (PVS); sadness does the opposite (Buck, 1999; Luu, Collins, & Tucker, 2000). Laughter is generated in the brainstem and is associated with the nucleus accumbens (Provine, 2001).

The medial forebrain is associated with the satisfaction of different drives and bodily needs, including hunger, thirst, sex, and temperature balance—and thus homeostasis and contentment. The lateral nucleus (LN) of the hypothalamus is associated with predatory joy, especially consumption—the anticipatory licking of the lips, the approach, and the pursuit. In the anterior and preoptic regions of the hypothalamus, joy comes when cries of distress are met with love and comfort. This area of the brain is rich in endogenous opiates (Hess, 1957).

Comfort releases endorphins. The septal region of the limbic system is important to joy, especially sexual joy. MacLean (1973) electrically stimulated the septal region of a female client's brain. In response, she stated, "I feel good. I have a glowing feeling."

The cingulate cortex is another area of the brain with a high concentration of opiate receptors. The thalamic cingulate region of the limbic system is central to playful fun and vocal communication associated with aggression and affiliative play.

Low amounts of monoamine oxidase, low naloxone, and low amounts of the neurotransmitter P coexist with a state of joy. It also is linked to high levels of endorphins, dopamine and norepinephrine, serotonin, gonadotropin-releasing hormone and oxytocin in women and vasopressin in men.

These positively associated neurohormones are a combination of stimulants and opiates.

Physiology and Joy

When we are in a state of joy, our mind is confident that it is a winner. The body is relaxed. Even when joy is aggressive, our body maintains a state of poise. Our happiness is associated with low heart rates, lower blood pressure, and lower levels of skin-conductance increases (less in happiness than in other emotions, with the exception of sadness and sleep [Vanderschuren, Niesink, & Van Ree, 1997]). Our muscle tension is usually low (with the exception of predatory joy [Panksepp, Siviy, & Normansell, 1984]). In fact, our body responds to joy and sadness similarly.

Joy tends to modulate stress. The neurohormone oxytocin, which is associated with joy, turns down the vigilance response triggered by the amygdala.

The Positives and Negatives of Joy

When we experience joy, we face many pitfalls. We can become arrogant when celebrating the joy of victory, as if we were the only participants who matter. Our joy becomes cruel when we rejoice in a victory that injures and humiliates others. Our joy becomes narcissism when victory is all about us. And our joy becomes denial when it blocks our vulnerable feelings of fear, sadness, and shame.

Buddha suggested that there were only two healthy expressions of joy. One was the joy in understanding, caring for, and having compassion for others. The other is the celebration of the victories of others. In Evelyn Loeb's collection of quotations about *Joy* (Loeb, 1991), she cites more reflections on *shared* joy than any other type of joy.

> All who would win joy must share it. Joy was born a twin.
>
> —Lord Byron

> Grief can take care of itself, but to get the full value of joy you must have somebody to divide it with.
>
> —Mark Twain

> It is a fine seasoning for joy to think of those we love.
>
> —Jean-Baptiste Molière

> A joy that's shared is a joy that's doubled.
>
> —English proverb

Who can enjoy alone, or, all enjoying, what contentment find?

—John Milton

Leaders of every major religion have taught that praising the Greater Power is the most healing and holy of all human activity. Perhaps this is true, whether the god be Buddha, Zoroaster, Yahweh, Mohammed, or Jesus. Praise that is transcendent and includes all of creation might be one of the most humbling and ennobling ways to experience joy. Feeling blessed, thankful, and praising a higher power might create a healthy, humbling, and loving psychological alignment.

Other joys are potentially healthy. There is the joy of the birth of a child, but that can sink into narcissism. The joy of creativity and the joy of mastery are not necessarily bad joys, but they easily escalate to conceit.

We can experience joy in shallow, narcissistic, and cruel ways. We can experience joy in healthy, inclusive, and gracious ways. But even though we know experiencing joy can be a positive happening, we don't want to be happy all the time.

By its very nature, life challenges us. Each of life's significant challenges will force us to fall down, be sad, ask for help, get angry, get back up, make a mistake, feel shame, make amends, feel fear, and learn from it, create an effective action plan, keep desire alive, stay motivated, achieve the goal, and feel the joy and satisfaction of accomplishment.

Yes, joy is the destination emotion. In sex, it is the climax. But as in sex, the journey, the anticipation, the planning, the uncertainty, and the excitement of desire are at least as important to the sexual experience as the climax. Once the climax is achieved, often we feel sad and lonely. Keeping the climax near without triggering its resolution is the advice of most sex-therapists.

The same is true for joy. "Joy," Armando Zegri, Chilean journalist and novelist, observed, "is a fruit that Americans eat green."

Happiness is not life's ultimate goal. Rather, living life to its fullest and feeling all the feelings life gives us is what makes life worth living. These are the accomplishments that will give us—and our clients—a rich and meaningful life.

Denial and Joy

Denial and repression are effective defenses against sadness and fear. Many of us refuse to feel these emotions and constantly display a happy smile on our faces.

In the musical *The King and I*, Anna sang to her frightened son, as their boat docked in the strange country of Siam.

In "Whistle a Happy Tune" (Richard Rodgers & Oscar Hammerstein II,1951) Anna tells her son that he can pretend to be happy by whistling a happy tune. He can use happiness and false bravado to fool not only those whom he fears but to fool himself as well. When he pretends to be happy he becomes convinced by his happy pose that he is not afraid.

Anna is right. This works. What we express in our faces triggers a biochemical event, releasing hormones that become a part of the body's expression of what our faces say to others that we feel. This pushes aside what we were feeling and replaces it with another feeling: in this case, the feeling is joy.

The only qualification that Ekman (1977) adds to this is that there is a crucial muscle around the eyes that must be moved to generate the physiology of happiness. If this muscle is not moved, the neurochemicals and neurocircuitry will not be turned on.

Even for those who limit their emotional expression to confident smiles, personal experiences can be so painfully dramatic that sadness, fear, surprise, and shame can break through momentarily only to be pushed quickly aside by a joke or a poised, practiced smile.

Is the joy that we maintain through repression and denial worth the cost? We therapists do not believe it is. So-called "dark" emotions have their place and need to be expressed. The world is not a safe place. When there is danger, we should feel fear. When we are mistreated, we should express anger to protect ourselves. Life is not paradise, and, when we think about it, we really don't want to be happy all the time. We want to feel all our emotions in response to daily challenges.

Joy signals that we are carefree, relaxed, and content. But in facing serious situations, we should react with a certain passion. We should care when our friend is hurt. We should be angry at injustice. We should develop drive and ambition that require hard work, risk, and sacrifice.

Individuals incapable of caring become sociopaths, happy and conscience-free. In the 1700s, King Ludwig of Prussia built several castles to imitate the grandeur of Versailles, taxing his people into poverty—and he didn't care. Marie Antoinette, in the face of her countrymen's poverty supposedly said, "Let them eat cake!" We don't want to help our clients become like Ludwig and Marie Antoinette. An emotional state of chronic joy creates a shallow and constricted person, and that's not the kind of person we—or our clients—should want to be.

Cruelty and Joy

A person who gains pleasure from his power over others is a tyrant; he is happy when he takes whatever he wants from others without caring, regretting, or feeling sad. This form of joy and constant happiness is cruel.

Think about film characters that represent evil. What expression do you see on their faces? What blood-curdling sounds do they make? The face smiles wickedly. With a cruel laugh the voice says, "Ah-ha-ha-ha! I'm about to eat you up!" Think of the twisted face of the Wicked Witch as she plots Snow White's death, or television's J.R. Ewing's delighted expression in the television show *Dallas* when he screws his brother Bobbie. Dylan Klebold and Eric Harris walked the halls of Columbine High School, laughing and shooting. These are portraits in evil. This is the dark side of joy.

Common expressions of this form of joy include: "I won;" "I'm the best;" "I'm number one;" "I'm the expert—the winner, the champion, the master;" "I have all the answers."

These also are expressions of dominance. In and of themselves, they pose no social problem. But they bring to mind other expressions: "I won, you lost." "I'm the best; you're inferior." "I'm number one; you're in last place." "I'm the expert; you're the novice." "I have all the answers; do what I tell you."

The Batterer and Self-Esteem

Research on family violence gives rise to debate: Does the person who batters have too much self-esteem? The batterer, like all bullies, does not have the strength to face sadness and failure. He insists on being the master who knows everything; he relegates other family members to sadness, fear, and shame—emotions the batterer himself refuses to feel (Stosny, 1995).

Those who suggest that the batterer has too much self-esteem might have confused the batterer's self-esteem with his demand that he be the one and only individual in the family who can feel joy. His inability to share joy with his family—to have the courage to feel sadness, fear, and shame—is in fact a consequence of low self-esteem.

To help families prevent violence, we professionals should teach the batterer that he can experience sadness, fear, and shame without personal disintegration and that his mate, too, has the right to win, know, be the expert, and experience joy.

Helping the young child move out of the role of bully calls on a similar procedure. Just as the batterer must first be afraid of the police and the courts, the young bully must be afraid of his or her parent or teacher.

After fear, sadness is the next emotion the bully must meet on the path toward a socially appropriate role. His sadness recognizes the loss of his dominant position; it is the natural consequence of letting go of that power. Shame, accountability, and honor follow sadness—all consequences of making amends and having compassion.

Wonder and Joy

Those who restrict themselves to joy by knowing it all or having all the answers miss a good portion of important meaningful human experience—the freedom and awe of the "not-knowing place." Many of us have difficulty accepting the vulnerable role of being empty, allowing others to fill us. There is great value in wonder, awe, mystery, and not knowing.

We need to help our clients, as well as ourselves, see the value of not knowing, the delight of wondering that is part of surprise, the deep commitment that is part of the sadness that comes from loving and losing, the honor that comes from shame, and the respect that is part of fear.

True self-esteem never comes from dominance over others. Rather, it comes from mastery over the self. Its basic ingredients include self-awareness, self-control, and ability to follow healthy emotional paths that use all the emotions.

Play and Joy

In our professional lives, we often encounter clients who long to achieve a state of joy. Here are lessons we can teach them.

In a struggle, you yearn for the happiness that achieving your goal will bring. The competition and teasing that is part of play can be mean, but it can also be a way to share in joy. Play should not be work; no real consequences are involved in play. Play should be a time of joyous abandon.

The Pretend Element

An important element of play is pretend. Pretending to be a brain surgeon is very different from operating on a brain. Pretending to take the last shot at the buzzer does not have the same significance as when Michael Jordan made a last-second three-pointer. Play uses our imagination and fantasies.

The Rules of Engagement

Play, when it involves others, requires that all players agree to play. It is not play if someone in the group is participating against her will. Someone forced to be part of an activity does not engage with the same enthusiasm, imagination, and desire as someone who chooses to participate. Forcing one's will on another ultimately provides little joy or pleasure. No one should be entitled to stand above the rules of the game. The rules of the game must apply equally to all players.

Successful play also requires respect. Participants need to feel that their respective roles are worthy of them. When players compete in a game, the game won't last long if the players aren't evenly matched and don't respect each other as potential worthy opponents.

The Cruelty Effect

Competition as play can become cruel if players and authorities are not careful. While it is true that joy most often has a competitive edge and that one who is capable of joy must relish a challenge, it is not true that the challenge must be personal.

The contest does not require hatred or an enemy. Often the challenge is to survive the ordeal of climbing a mountain; master the skill of drawing a flower; or defeat entropy by creating a beautiful space; discover harmony by learning to perform on an instrument in an ensemble; reach the best level of play against a worthy opponent.

Often contests present adversaries. This situation brings with it the temptation to make the opponent the enemy, an act often accompanied by cruelty and hatred. When the contest becomes personal, pain is a natural consequence of playing. This is why some people do not enjoy sports that pit one contestant against another. Instead, they enjoy contests against the elements, such as skiing down a mountain where the adversary is gravity and the object is to stay upright.

Competing against one another can be an exciting challenge. But our task is to focus on the contest as a way to discover the best in us as competitors. Events such as the America's Cup, Superbowl, Wimbledon, or the state championship, encourage participants to concentrate on the event and to view other contestants as obstacles who will test their skills. The prize is not the vanquishing of a specific person. The trophy symbolizes victory.

The Role of Sharing

To be a healthy winner, participants must avoid arrogance. We must share our victory with other participants—the support team, the organizers, and the audience. In sharing our victory, we will safely experience joy.

The most dramatic moments are self-made. We take on the contest, not because we have to, but because we want to. When we win, we have the opportunity to experience joy. But it is in losing that we learn how to improve. Winning gives no guidance. We have no model to help teach us how to better our performance. When we lose, we can see what we need to do to improve by contrasting our skills with winners. Losing can bring with it the gift of knowledge. And, after all, it is just a game.

To protect play, remember four points:

1. This is just a game, meaning this is pretend. There are no real consequences for what happens here, and there will be another game another time.
2. The rules of the game must be known by all players and must apply to all participants equally.
3. Play involves challenge, but the challenge need not be personal. Play need not create an enemy.
4. The best challenge is to play to beat our own best, play against the other to bring out the best in us, play against the course, field, or challengers as worthy opponents. This minimizes loss and prevents our joy from becoming cruelty.

When We Win, We Lose

If we hoard the credit for our accomplishments, victories, and successes, we will eventually cut ourselves off from our support network. Others won't join our team. People won't trust us as collaborators. No one will invite us to participate.

The winner of a marathon should acknowledge the people who put water out along the route, the people who shouted encouragement along the way, the people who trained with her and helped her with her daily routine of eating right, exercising, and getting rest, her opponents who helped her find her best.

Sharing the joy of an accomplishment brings pride to a whole community, and the community will always celebrate the winner as its representative, as its champion.

Humor and Joy

"The closer we get to understanding what makes us laugh, the further we get from humor" (Johnson, 2004, p. 117). Provine (2001) suggests the incongruity theory of humor/laughter occurs when you are expecting one thing and you get another. Surprise is followed by relief. Johnson (2004) reports the results of a study of humor by a British research group. Its members purport to have discovered the world's funniest joke. It goes like this:

> A couple of New Jersey hunters are out in the woods when one of them falls to the ground. He doesn't seem to be breathing; his eyes are rolled back in his head. The other guy whips out his cell phone and calls emergency services. He gasps to the operator: "My friend is dead! What can I do?"
>
> The operator, in a calm, soothing voice, says: "Just take it easy. I can help. First, let's make sure he's dead." There is silence, then a shot

is heard. The guy's voice comes back on the line. He says: "OK, now what?"

The context set up in the joke creates the expectation that the hunter on the phone will check his comrade's pulse. The surprise is that he shoots the hunter instead. We laugh because it is unexpected and because it is not us lying on the ground. We are pleased that the surprise didn't create fear in us.

Therapists must explain to their clients that laughter is partially dark. We all laugh when someone is humiliated when slipping on a banana peel. Such ridicule is an exchange of self-esteem. The person ridiculed is humiliated, and her self-esteem is lost. The person laughing feels superior and takes the self-esteem from the person who slipped and fell. As Mark Twain wrote, "The secret source of humor is not joy but sorrow." An amendment to Twain's quote might be "and the fact that the sorrow is not ours."

Teasing is a form of humor. It is behavior that appears to be tormenting and cruel, but isn't. Teasing is a form of play that presumes upon the goodwill and friendship of another. Teasing can include rough play, tickling, or pulling a pigtail. The tease becomes play when the seemingly cruel behavior is viewed as a challenge to play, not as an attempt to intimidate or hurt. Teasing triggers the startle response. The amygdala fires, waking up the body and preparing for threat. When the assumption of threat is tested and proved wrong, joy and laughter are the result. The body is relieved of its duty to fight or run. The body is alert, safe, and relieved.

Avoiding Cruelty

How can we tell funny stories without becoming a cruel jokester and smart aleck? Humor that consistently is funny occurs when we laugh at ourselves. No one is sufficiently informed, equipped, and prepared for life's twists and turns. Life is full of surprises. It helps to see humor in life and in the human condition. When we can call on our sense of humor as we face life's challenges, we become a treasure.

The slip and fall on a banana peel can have a kinder side. Laughter can come from a surprise or startling event (for example, suddenly being upended by a slippery banana peel) that turns out well, when no one is hurt. Laughter is the relief and the celebration of victory over the potentially dangerous surprise. If the individual who slips can laugh at her own predicament, she creates a communal joyful moment, giving permission to all present to laugh along with her, volunteering herself as the butt of the joke.

Most humor is cruel and has a victim. Jay Leno's and David Letterman's late-night monologues attest to this. No subject or individual is immune from their stinging verbal jabs.

At times, we might have enjoyed humiliating others. For example, child-hood is a time of building power and competence. We are sensitive about what we are not yet able to do as a child and often compensate for our inadequacy by making fun of the others' inadequacies. (You might remember, as a child, laughing at someone whose face was scarred, who walked with a limp, or who had seizures—calling them monsters, or worse.)

When someone sets out intentionally to do harm, our rational response is to be offended. But in the spirit of play, we are not offended when others poke fun at us if we recognize that sometimes we act and look pretty silly. We can use these moments to laugh at ourselves and to play with others. Humor redeems failure and gives us joy in the face of tragedy.

Entertainment and Joy

Joy comes when there is an increased challenge or demand for attention, followed by a sudden decrease in this demand or challenge. Good times are characterized by shifts from increased demands for vigilance, followed by relief that the danger has passed.

Watch a father tickling his young daughter. His hands challenge her to defend herself against what seems to be tormenting tickling. Then, he with-draws his hands when she says, "Stop!" Feeling safe and joyful, she laughs and runs away. Sometimes, she will come back to him, inviting him to repeat the tickling—and he does.

The fun has increase of stimuli, followed by decrease—a sort of crescendo and diminuendo of activity. This increase and decrease is not so intense as to be out of bounds. The individual's expected set of behaviors is not so chal-lenged that these playful actions become serious or frightening.

An intense increase in the challenge presented by the tickling father can push the limits of predictability—the daughter is afraid for a moment. Her fear dissipates when the father decreases the tickling, thus withdrawing the challenge.

The Components of Entertainment

Entertainment comprises three parts:

1. Tension or challenge in order to set up the pattern of increase in stimuli;
2. Boundaries that are pushed but not broken;
3. Conclusion, ending with a relieving decrease in stimuli.

This means entertainment can challenge. It contains elements of fear, respect, and cruelty. It has just enough characteristics of cruelty to raise the question, "Am I safe here?", followed by the reassuring moment that rees-tablishes a sense of well-being and safety. The answer to the safety question then becomes, "Yes, I am safe." Joy follows this answer.

Fear must be touched and relieved as we are entertained. The more your client is able to believe that she can handle the challenge of fear in play, the more she will have the courage to face real fear and to conquer it.

Pride and Joy

Pride is the kind of joy we feel when we have accomplished a challenging goal. Of course, we think that we want to be proud of ourselves, but do we really?

Pride's Two Faces

There are two kinds of pride: healthy and false. Healthy pride comes from a job well done, an effort that brings out the best in us. We deserve to be proud of hard work, delayed gratification, sacrifice, practice, discipline, followed by success. We want our clients to have enough of these experiences, and of rewards resulting from their best efforts, so that they have pride in who they are and faith in themselves. They need this to have healthy self-esteem. And so do we.

Pride that comes from the pleasure of defeating another, or from the joy of being special, entitled, or better than another, is false pride. It is not based on hard work and achievement but on the status that comes from beauty, luck, or popularity. We can't depend on luck, personal attractiveness, or the whimsical likes and dislikes of others. While genuine healthy pride always supports us, false pride always betrays us.

Real joy, believe me, is a serious matter.

—Seneca (1963)

Innocence and Joy

Often the experience of joy can include a sense of entitlement, specialness, and "better-thanness." Joy can create traps that impale our character. It is difficult for any of us to find politically correct humor or joy without some degree of narcissism. Does that mean that we should not allow ourselves to feel impure joy?

If joy leads to play, learning, and love, it must bring some good—even if some bad tags along. Too often girls in our culture are taught to avoid the celebration of victory if the victory means that someone else must feel the pain of defeat. Some people never laugh at a joke, because they always see that it hurts the object of the humor, even when the object of the humor also enjoys the laugh at her own expense.

Joyful moments are precious. We should encourage them. We should try to forgive ourselves and others when joy is less than perfect. We should encourage our clients to feel joy when they can and hope that joy will open them to learning, love, and compassion for others.

Shame and Joy

In chapter 10, we discuss the special relationship between shame and joy—examining it under the light of shame needing resolution. Here, we focus on that relationship with joy as our focus.

The Role of Humor

Because joy and shame are so naturally related, we often use humor or laughter on the front end of shame. This laughter indicates, "I know I did something foolish, but I don't have to feel bad about it, do I?" If the individual that we might have harmed laughs too, we assume shame is not required of us. This illustrates embarrassed laughter.

Laughter at the misfortune of others makes a similar statement. It means, "I am so relieved. That could have been me. I'm glad it wasn't." This joy is associated with potential shame and hurt that fate gave to someone else instead of to us.

Often we take a playful jab at a friend and follow our jest with laughter, as if to say we enjoy the privilege of being able to tease our good friend this way. This privilege is confirmed by our friend's wry smile that says to us, "No, I won't require you to feel ashamed for what you said, because I know we are friends."

Shame and Sex

Then, there is the joy of sex. Shame is the primary inhibitor of the sexual impulse (Nathanson, 1992). To make a sexual initiative, we must first overcome the potential shame of rejection. Overcoming our fears of shame—and avoiding the contempt and disgust that the object of our desire might express—are great achievements and part of the pleasure of sexual consummation.

Resolving Joy

The Let-Down Effect

Your clients might well ask, "Why would I want to resolve joy?" Joy as an emotion often resolves itself into boredom/relaxation.

Often, after we have completed climbing our personal mountain, we experience confusion and depression. We have lost our life's organizing principle and sense of direction. Before our success, we had a way of prioritizing decisions simply by looking at the next step toward our goal. With this goal achieved, we might not know what to do with ourselves. We can only celebrate so long. If we don't have an answer to "So, what now," we risk becoming lost.

When joy moves to boredom, boredom moves us to look for a new challenge or interest. This new goal can create all the other emotions of fear, anger, sadness, shame, surprise, and disgust.

Mired in Joy

Though healthy joy has a standard pattern of resolving itself (for example, joy—boredom—interest/excitement) some individuals refuse to leave the state of joy and contentment. They can become smug, arrogant bullies. Their joy needs to be resolved for their sakes and certainly for ours.

Rarely does a therapist face the task of helping people stuck in joy move beyond their joy. Why would such a person come to therapy? Such a person could be a court-ordered batterer or a teenager who rules and controls her parents. These individuals have no incentive to change. Change would mean that they would lose power. Change would require that they share self-esteem and joy instead of hoarding it for themselves. Change would mean that they would have to face the fears that can overwhelm them when they face the reality that they don't know.

I will treat the batterer who is afraid of going to jail, because he has the incentive to learn and to cooperate with treatment (see chapter 5, anger). But I won't treat the teenager who is controlling a family. Instead, I treat the teenager's parents. These parents must give their child a reason to change, and that reason is fear. Fear creates the respect parents must have to regain their authority.

Fear, of course, is the first socializing emotion. Possibly compassion will later replace it. Children and adults always worry about the feelings of others, if those others are bigger, stronger, and angry because of what they did or said. Fear takes away our joy—cruel or otherwise.

Confronting Cruel Joy

Shame is especially important in resolving cruel joy (see chapter 10). The client who can say, "I'm sorry," followed by "I know what I did, and it was wrong," is on the way toward healing relationships and salving wounds inflicted by the arrogance of her cruel joy. Sadness that her pleasure hurt someone is also a useful antidote to cruel joy. Fear that she might do this again becomes motivation to change. The respect that comes from fear helps her learn compassion. Compassion helps the client include others' feelings in her problem-solving so that she is no longer able to enjoy the pain of another.

The courts and other authorities use fear to help our clients move beyond cruel joy. Although sometimes fear must be the first emotion our clients feel, it is not the only emotion we want for our clients as they emerge from the arrogance of cruel joy. We hope our clients will learn respect and compassion from their fear.

The Therapist's Job

Put aside your anger and disgust. As a therapist, your job is not to frighten or to shame your client. If you remain angry and use your anger and disgust to resolve your client's cruel joy into shame, your client will imitate your behavior and learn to entitle her anger and disgust when she perceives others as in the wrong.

Anger only empowers cruelty. Anger brings with it the two-category thinking of enemy/ally and a sense of entitlement that convinces us that we have a right to our predatory cruelty.

In addition to the challenge of managing our anger for the client, we must help her avoid fear as her destination emotion. When we leave our client in fear, we create an anxious, fearful individual who will have difficulty developing trusting relationships.

Sadness and Shame

The emotions that leave the most honorable legacy are first, sadness, and second, shame. Between these two, sadness is my first choice.

When an individual is sad that others are in pain, she is in the first stage of compassion. Compassion always gives us memories we can be proud of, while anger or joy in the pain of others alienates us from our community, friends, and family, as well as cuts us off from those we consider enemies. Compassion opens doors and reconnects adversaries.

The second, shame, is difficult for any of us, perhaps especially our clients, to negotiate. It takes courage to feel badly when we acknowledge a mistake. After your client has used shame to resolve cruel joy, help your client to be proud that she can say, "I'm sorry," take responsibility, and feel shame. This helps improve relationships and makes amends that potentially can right wrongs. Shame used this way is an important social resource.

Your client has earned the right to be pleased with the capacity shame has given her to heal relationships.

Survival and Joy

Nico Frijda (1986) contends that joy gives the body vague behavioral instructions associated with aimless activity. Certainly joy does not provide the same specific instructions that our more negative emotions do (for example, fear tells us to flee, anger to fight, shame to cease and desist, sadness to let go). The messages that come from negative emotions are essential to our survival. But positive emotions appear, at first glance, to have inconsequential effects on our survival.

In her book *The Broaden and Build Theory of Positive Emotions* (2001), Barbara Fredrickson answers this challenge. She contends that there are five positive emotions: joy, interest, contentment, pride, and love. She also mentions gratitude (McCullough, Kilpatrick, Emmons, & Larson, 2001) and elevation (Haidt, 2000).

My model of emotions disagrees with Fredrickson's (2001). In my model, her list would be reduced to two basic emotions: joy and interest. Contentment and pride are derivatives of joy. Love is a complex set of behaviors that involves several emotions. Her model implies that there are negative emotions. In my view, all emotions can be positive. But that is being unfairly critical of Fredrickson. Even if we use the more neutral terms—light emotions and dark emotions—we might still quibble with Fredrickson about some of her choices.

For us, *joy* is the only, clearly positive basic emotion. Even then, we suggest that joy has a dark side. Interest can reflect "I want to approach," making it light, as well as "I want to avoid," making it dark.

Although I would consider *interest* a basic emotion, I believe it would be more accurately considered a neutral emotion along with surprise/startle/wonder.

Contentment is certainly a light emotion, but it is not a pure basic emotion as is joy. Rather it is a combination of joy and the trance. It says, "I am safe, relaxed, and happy."

Pride is an expression derived from joy. It is a combination of positive cognitive self-evaluation and joy. It has emotional and personal judgment components: the happiness that comes from a history of success and the confidence that comes from a cognitive prediction of future successes. Pride says, "I am competent," "I can, I know, and I will," "Look at me. I just did that. Hooray!"

Love is a complex emotion. It contains the potential of shame if we harm someone we love. It has the joy of communion, mutual sharing, and acceptance. It also has an interest/excitement component. And it has the peace and safety that comes from the trance.

Fredrickson suggests that each of these emotions has an important species-adaptive function. Each broadens our perspective and builds positive coping skills.

"*Joy*," she writes, "broadens by creating the urge to play, push the limits, and be creative. These urges are evident not only in social and physical behavior but also in intellectual and artistic behavior" (p. 220). The creative play that comes from joy evolves into practice that evolves into new skills (for example, new dance steps, new songs, new moves to the hoop).

"*Interest*...broadens by creating the urge to explore, take in new information and experiences, and expand the self in the process" (p. 220). New information can stimulate new ideas; new ways to problem-solve and improve planning. Certainly these skills are relevant to our survival.

"*Contentment*," she continues, "broadens by creating the urge to savor current life circumstances and integrate these circumstances into new views of the self and of the world" (ibid., p 220). Contentment encourages reflection. It helps us see what it is that we did that worked, so that we can repeat it when the situation warrants. Psychologists know that we help children most by calling attention to the good they do, praising them, giving them a moment of contentment for safe reflection.

"*Pride*...broadens by creating the urge to share news of achievements with others and to envision even greater achievement in the future" (ibid., p. 220). Pride gives us the courage and confidence to risk. Pride helps us get up and try again or try something different after we have fallen. The confidence that comes from pride keeps us from giving up. It gives us the survivor spirit.

"*Love*...broadens by creating recurring cycles of urges to play with, explore, savor experiences with loved ones (and) envision future achievements (with loved ones)" (ibid., p. 220). Love gives us the urge to protect one another, to confirm that we are safe together to play, explore, risk, and savor. Love creates an atmosphere of acceptance that inoculates us from the toxicity that can come from the negative emotions of anger, shame, and sadness. It is well documented that social support (love) aids survival.

In her book, Fredrickson also contends that positive emotions make us more resilient. They give us the confidence that a resilient person needs to reframe events in ways that give new opportunities to problem-solve, rather than give up. Positive emotions help us stay creatively problem-focused rather than surrendering to negative, introverted self-appraisals. Positive emotions give us faith that somehow, if we keep looking, we will find good and success will follow.

Just as there are well-documented, negative spirals that have a defeating and depressing downward momentum, there are also upward spirals that are triggered by positive emotions. Positive emotions help us find positive meaning in life's minutiae and even in painful experience. Finding positive meaning in adversity creates positive emotions, and positive emotions help us find positive reframes.

Practiced over time, the skill of finding positive meaning in adversity builds and accumulates just like any other skill.

"The broadened attention and cognition triggered by earlier experiences of positive emotion should facilitate coping with adversity, and this improved coping should predict future experiences of positive emotion. As this cycle continues, people build their psychological resilience and enhance their emotional well being.... The broaden-and-build theory predicts a comparable upward spiral, in which positive emotions and the broadened (creative) thinking they engender also influence one another reciprocally, leading to appreciable increases in emotional well-being over time" (ibid., p. 223).

While I might differ with Fredrickson about definitions and while I would warn of the dangerous traps in joy, I am certainly persuaded by Fredrickson's research and theory. Joy is essential to our survival. Learning, growing, and developing new skills does not happen easily when we are afraid, sad, ashamed, or angry. Joy can create the atmosphere for love, effective growth, and development.

Ritual to Help Us Become More Emotionally Aware

A State of Cool

In the minds of adolescents, being unfeeling, being impervious to fear, sadness, anger, or shame are termed being "cool," or what might be called false contentment. This is a highly desirable state for many young people. Boys especially are taught not to feel weak, tender feelings. We throw a football at them and tell them to catch it and run straight toward 11 other boys who intend to bury them. The point of this tribal initiation is to teach boys to perform in the face of fear, to learn not to feel fear or sadness or shame, and instead to use repression, denial, and anger to help them perform.

A State of Contemplation

Adults often use false contentment as a badge of faith, religious and otherwise. Faith is the antidote to fear. "If we believe, how could we not be happy" is a rational for avoiding what we really feel. This false contentment, termed faith, is justification for what psychologists term alexathymia, or "not being aware" of what we feel. Once we become practiced at the posture of false contentment (or always answering the question, "How are you?" with "I am fine"), we don't know how to get out of this unfeeling trap.

Many adults recognize that they would prefer to feel and use all their feelings rather than be trapped in false contentment.

Following is a ritual that can build emotional awareness in our clients and help them begin to know and use their feelings effectively. It is an acronym using the letters of HELP to represent the four steps to emotional awareness.

 Step 1: Happy, really? Instead of saying "I'm fine" or "I'm happy," say to yourself, "I don't know how I feel. And that is just one of the many things I don't know." Be curious about yourself. What feelings might you be covering with false contentment? Search your heart for feelings of fear (we always have reason to fear) or sadness, or shame, or doubt, or yearning, or disgust.

 Step 2: Engage these vulnerable feelings when you find them. Feel them instead of covering them up. Admit to yourself what you feel. Express these feelings aloud to someone else or in writing to yourself.

 Step 3: Let somebody help you. Admit you don't know. Ask for help. Admit that you need someone else's energy, strength, ideas, or companionship. Let somebody love you. Asking for help is the victory. But do not expect that you will receive help just because you ask for it. Yours is a request, not a command. Asking for help does not entitle you to control another. Be prepared to go without help. Ask, however, and you might receive. If you don't, help may not come. Your achievement is in the asking. So keep asking.

 Step 4: Prepare for a new challenge. Gather your forces. Accept what help you can get. Begin your next adventure. Proceed, using your real feelings instead of pretending that you don't feel them.

Summary and Conclusion

Remember Howard and Virginia at the beginning of this chapter? Virginia's final response to Howard provides a summary statement for this chapter. We pick up where Howard said, "The reason I won't give you a diamond is that it won't make any difference. You will just want something else next week, and I can't do anything that would make you happy."

Virginia replied, "I'm not for sale."

"What does that mean?" Howard asked. "Who's trying to buy you?"

"You are, Howard. You want to buy me something to shut me up, that will put a permanent smile on my face and transform me into a sexy French maid who is waiting for the master to come home. When he does, she will ooze happiness and gratitude all over him, as she takes off his shoes, puts on his slippers, listens to him relate his heroics, and then takes him to bed. Well, Howard, I am a person, too. I am not some whore whom you can make happy with money.

"Sure," Virginia continued, "I want to be happy. But I don't want to be happy because of you. I want a life. I'm not just your wife. I have a right to challenges that scare me. I have a right to feel anxious and frightened, sad, embarrassed, surprised, tired, angry, all those feelings. I have a right to feel without feeling guilty. In fact, I want to feel all these ways. Don't you?"

"No," was Howard's curt reply.

"Well, I'm sorry for you," Virginia went on. "I want to be the hero of my own story, not a handmaiden in yours. This means I will have lots of feelings. If this makes me an unhappy demanding bitch in your eyes, divorce me, Howard."

"I don't want a divorce. That's why we are here," Howard insisted.

"Well, Howard, you are right. I have tagged along with your life looking to you to make me happy. The only time I felt fulfilled was when I had our children to care for. But even then I wasn't happy all the time. If I just wanted to be happy, I would sit on the beach drinking tequila all day. That would make me happy. But that's not what I want. Why am I not entitled to a challenge of my own? Why does my happiness always have to come from you?

"I will never be just happy, Howard. You are right, and you will never make me happy. I'm sorry that I ever let either of us think that my happiness would come from you or that joy was what I wanted. I want meaning to my life more than anything else. You are off the hook. I will take responsibility for my emotions from now on. I wish you could feel something other than 'fine,' Howard. I'm sorry you can't or won't.'"

"Okay, Doctor. I accept that challenge," Howard responded. "Tell me what to do to feel something other than 'fine.' I'll do whatever it takes to make her happy, but I don't know what I can do about being too happy."

"Well, try this ritual Howard," I said. "Do it at least once a day or more and see if you begin to feel different, more aware of other feelings that you always felt, but perhaps didn't acknowledge. Maybe that will help you make deeper emotional connections with Virginia. And come back alone weekly for a while, and let's see how things go."

Howard did as I asked. He used the HELP ritual. After 6 weeks, he said, "I don't know why I'm more aware of how I feel. I think I was afraid to feel. I needed the practice. That ritual you gave me allowed me to try on different feelings for size, and I did. It wasn't so bad. Sadness didn't capture me. I felt sad for a while, then I bounced back.

"I had been feeling shame a long time, because I didn't seem to be able to make Virginia happy and I feel shame about a lot of things. I guess I felt shame and covered it, pretending to know things and be happy. I was angry at Virginia for being so demanding and not being happy, but my anger was just a cover for my fear and shame. I think I am always a little bit afraid, but ashamed to admit it. Now that I think about it, when I wrote my first book, I was frightened and felt inadequate to the task at the beginning. I almost called my editor and quit. As I wrote, I would get excited about getting something down on paper, and then I would feel lost again. When it was published, I was afraid it would not be well received. And I was sad when it didn't become a best-seller.

"When I recently told this to Virginia, she said she felt closer to me knowing this. We talk more. She seems to enjoy it when I tell her about the negative feelings I'm discovering. She says she doesn't feel so alone or so much like a bitch now. And I'm less afraid of her feelings, as I get more comfortable with my own. Several times I've asked Virginia to help me or teach me or help me think about something, and she has been able to most of the time. That has felt good to both of us. I guess it's OK not to be master of the universe."

CHAPTER 9

Interest/Desire/Excitement[9]
The Emotions' Source of Positive Energy

Interest/Desire/Excitement Defined

According to Lorenz (1950), "interest typically occurs in pattern with joy." Interest enlivens and excites. It motivates the approach response and supplies the drive that pushes us toward meeting our survival needs. This is Freud's libido. Because interest represents drive, it is a modulated emotion. It has a range and that range is part of its essence. It is not just on or off. It moves from mild interest to desire, to strong desire, to frantic excitement.

According to Tomkins (1962), interest is the force that allows us to sustain long-term creative and constructive endeavors. It keeps us connected to our environment and, together with contentment, is one of our emotional steady states. These states can last a long time, although other emotions may intrude and interrupt them.

Interest organizes our focus of attention to stimuli. If we are hungry, for example, interest blocks other stimuli and focuses our attention on food. Novel stimuli provoke interest (Fetterman, 1996). Interest helps us maintain our homeostasis when a lot is happening around us. The new stimulus excites us so that we attend to it, until we clearly understand how that stimulus relates to our survival. If we find it is irrelevant, we ignore it and attend to things that we believe will better serve us.

Interest is the emotion that alerts our body and individuals around us that we are approaching something we want to have or consume. Most of the time, we consider it a positive emotion. But we sometimes forget that interest comes from our biological appetites. It is part of gluttony, greed, envy, jealousy, lust for power, sex, and fame. With the exception of anger, these "I-wants" can get us in more trouble than any other emotion.

Excitement is an enthusiastic response that expresses how intensely we want to consume, hold, and possess something that is near. Excitement includes anticipation of the pleasure of consumption and fear that we won't get what we want. Interest, excitement, and desire are different parts of the same emotion—the difference between them is simply a matter of intensity and focus. Excitement is the equivalent of intense interest. Desire identifies an object that is our focus. Interest is the steady state of paying attention and being on task.

Clinical Case Study

I was seeing Craig. A prominent and well-respected divorce attorney, known as one of the best litigators and negotiators in town, he was caught in a love triangle.

"People think I'm a great lawyer and problem solver," Craig explained, "and maybe I am for other people. But I just can't seem to solve my problems or, more specifically, this problem. My wife, Enid, and I had been designing our dream house for years. I was making good money. We both agreed that we would save enough to pay for the house before it was built. I realized that we would still probably have to borrow—you know how construction costs can expand. We had met with the architect several times. We had a building lot on top of a hill that overlooks the city.

"I wanted to give Enid this house in the worst way," he continued. "I invested our savings in stocks. I had a chance to get some ADW Net at $18 when it came out as an initial public offering. I bet all of our savings on it, and I bought some more on the margin, using our lot as equity.

"If there was ever a sure thing this was it. The week it came out, ADW Net went up from $18 to $24. Later it got to $36. Just a little more, and I could pay for the house and then some. Enid knew nothing about this.

"Well, you know what's coming," Craig predicted. "The stock fell and fell. The brokerage firm called in my margin account. I had to sell our lot. I needed Enid's signature for that. When I told her, she was shocked, enraged. Disappointment wasn't even close to how she felt. From that day on, I have not been able to look at her straight in the face. I feel indescribable guilt.

"About one month after I lost my dream home with Enid, Lindsay came to ask me to represent her in her divorce from Carl Davenport, the richest man in Nashville. This was a complicated case. Lindsay and I had to spend a great deal of time together going through tax returns and investment portfolios. We had to take trips together to visit various warehouses and real estate holdings that she and Carl owned. Of course, Carl didn't feel that she owned any of it. In the trial, the judge agreed with me that Lindsay owned one-half of the whole estate, over $200,000,000.

"To Enid, I was a goat. To Lindsay, I was a hero. Well, I couldn't look at Enid, and I couldn't take my eyes off of Lindsay. She was vulnerable to my attention. Before long, Lindsay and I became lovers. I was sure Enid was so disgusted with me that she would be glad to get rid of me. I told her that I thought she should divorce me. I was shocked when she responded that my idea was the stupidest thing she ever heard me say. She loved me. We had suffered disappointments, but life is full of those. She was my partner for better or worse. Losing our house was part of the worse. The better, she said, would come back. Time would heal.

"'Part of the better,' she said, 'was our children.' They are both teenagers. Craig, Jr., is a senior in high school. Margaret is in the ninth grade. They are great kids. They are definitely part of the better. Enid is right. We are married, partners in good times and bad. I want that.

"And I want Lindsay, too. I know I should leave Lindsay. I go to her apartment to tell her. I walk in the door, into her adoring eyes looking at me as her champion returned from the wars. She wraps me up in her kisses, and then I leave Lindsay with the resolve to tell Enid that I want a divorce. I walk in the door at home and see the portrait over the fireplace of the four of us, and I know I want to be home with my family.

"I want so much, so much that I can't have. I can't stop wanting what I want. I don't have the strength to give up, either Enid or Lindsay. I want to stop all this wanting. I will do whatever it takes. Please help me," Craig pleaded. "I no longer can trust myself."

The Neurology of Interest/Desire/Excitement

Interest includes circuits that are also used in other emotions. The amygdala, primarily associated with fear and anger, is specifically connected to the olfactory circuitry, thus making the amygdala key to stimulating the hunger drive (Teitelbaum, 1961).

Also connected to the olfactory circuits in the brain is the septal region, important to stimulating the sex drive. Yet a third circuit—the thalamocingulate—stimulates the desire for affiliation and acceptance. This circuit includes the mammillothalmic tract, which connects these to the anterior thalamus and then to the cingulate gyrus. This circuit, in turn, connects to the visual, audiovocal tracts (Panksepp, 1993).

In the brainstem, the ascending reticular-activating system (ARAS) produces electroencephaloghic arousal and alerting (Lindsley, 1951). The ARAS controls two types of arousal (Lindsley, 1957). The first is more cholinergic, using primarily acetylcholine (ACH). It stimulates voluntary purposive behavior that requires input from other parts of the brain. The second type of arousal consists of more primitive responses, for example, vocalization, ejaculation, urination, and defecation. The ARAS serves as a stimulus filter, focusing the brain and the body only on the relevant stimuli while ignoring the rest (Bremer, 1935). Examples of this are selective attending and tunnel vision.

The medial forebrain bundle (MFB) is particularly associated with the appetite. This part of the hypothalamus directs us to the environmental incentives, for example, food, water, sex partners, and coolness or warmth (Teitelbaum, 1961).

The main neurohormones associated with interest/excitement/desire are dopamine and norepinephrine. Together with other amines, these regulate the speed of mental activity, attention, and awareness (Panksepp, 1981).

Interest/desire/excitement is negatively related to monoamine oxidase and, of course, the pain peptide, substance P. Many other hormones that are associated with fear or pleasure, for example, will also function to focus and stimulate interest. They include glutamate and pentapeptide leu-enkephalin.

The Physiology of Interest/Desire/Excitement

Since this emotion ranges from the steady state of mild interest to the high-energy state of excitement, we have difficulty pinpointing how this emotion affects the body. This depends on where in the range this emotion exists. This fact used to disqualify interest/desire/excitement as an emotion. But those who eliminate arousal completely prevent us from understanding this primarily dimensional emotion that is more complex than just being "on" or "off."

The Intelligence of Interest/Desire/Excitement

Recently, the desire for the things we think will make us happy has been the subject of a great deal of research. The primary researchers in this area are a team of psychologists and economists. They are Tom Gilbert, a Harvard psychologist; Tim Wilson, a psychologist from the University of Virginia; George Lowenstein, an economist at Carnegie Mellon; and Dan Kahneman, a psychologist and Nobel laureate in economics. They collectively discovered that we are not very smart about our interests. The things we want, the things we believe will make us happy, do not. Their findings mirror Mark Twain's famous sarcastic statement, "Beware of what you want for you shall surely get it." Gilbert and Wilson (2000) found that we overestimate our emotional reaction to things we believe we want. When we get them, they suddenly seem to lose their value for us. They call this "impact bias," meaning our tendency toward the bias of overestimating the impact value of things we want. Our desires have poor judgment. Some of us may think consummating a relationship will make us happy. We find that once we have what we wanted, we don't want it anymore. These mistakes in our expectation of our desired goal to make us happy can direct us to things that make us miserable. For example, we may wish to marry a sexually oriented mate only to find that our mate doesn't contain his or her sexual interest just to us. We may want a new car, but cannot afford the car payment. The problem is not what the Rolling Stones say: "You can't always get what you want!" It is that what we want is often not what we need.

What happens in our brains, according to Lowenstein (1999), is that we adapt to the thing that once made us happy. When we achieved our goal, it was a new experience for us. But once it becomes a part of our normal life, it loses its allure for us. It becomes part of the context of our lives. Most of the time we do not realize this, as we are focusing on the object of our desire. We do not know that our desire has this flaw and that we will not find happiness where or how we think we will.

Another problem about the human process of wanting and desiring is that when we imagine ourselves getting what we think we want, when we get there, the experience is nothing like we imagined. A terminally ill woman with gastro-intestinal problems imagined that she would eat and enjoy a banana pie. When she got a piece of banana pie, she could not find her desire. This is what Lowenstein calls the "empathy gap." In addition to the empathy gap and impact bias, we tend not to learn from our mistakes. We forget the pain of a circumstance and only remember the joy. This is a mother's experience of childbirth. According to Lowenstein, our desires and the desiring process does not seem to learn from experience.

The Negative Consequences of Interest/Desire/Excitement

A parent's greatest joy is to satisfy a child's wants. Certainly, parents are pleased that their children have a personality that expresses their unique desires. And parents should be pleased when their children clearly express their needs and wants in their interest and excitement.

But problems occur when, in a common environment, children desire the same object. Indeed, this problem occurs also when adults compete for the same resources.

Interest/desire/excitement is the emotional base of words like: want, greed, lust, envy, gluttony, and passion. What happens when our "I-wants" become obsessive, and we won't be satisfied until we get what we can't have? We become frustrated. These frustrations are part of our everyday existence. These "I-wants" become the basis of parental/child power struggles. They are the basis of our struggle with ourselves. Children's "I want, I want, I want, I want . . ." exhausts and confuses parents and other adults.

But our own desires can be more confusing. We often don't know what to do with interest. We can't seem to satisfy our children. We don't know how to respond to a child who, as soon as she is given one thing, quickly wants another. Just as we can become slaves to our child's desires, we can become a slave to our own "I-wants."

In the emotion of interest/desire/excitement, we develop our character. Here, we answer the question: Can we control ourselves, or do our impulses control us? If we cannot trust ourselves to act in our own best interest, it follows that others cannot trust us. Interest/desire/excitement continues to try us. We can fall prey to the various addictions—drugs, sex, even addiction to joy and anger. Or, we can learn the skills of telling the difficult truth to ourselves and others, denying our immediate desires for our overall best interests and for those of our community and family, thus delaying our wants until fulfilling them is not harmful to others or ourselves.

Clients with addictions need help. They find that they cannot fight their wants alone. Their desires become emotional obsessions. Their attention becomes fixated on one object of desire. It might be a work project. It might be drugs. It might be exercise, food, or sex. Their attention can become fixated on a single thing, and there is never enough of that one thing to satisfy them. Seemingly, the client's drive toward a goal cannot be satiated even when she achieves this goal. In addiction, she experiences no real joy. And perhaps that's the problem.

Delay of Gratification

In the 1960s, Walter Mischel and Phillip Peake conducted a now-famous longitudinal study of 4-year-olds. They offered each of their subjects two options: a treat of one marshmallow now, or a treat of two marshmallows later if they could wait for the marshmallows until the researcher returned from running errands. This procedure created two groups—one that could not delay gratification and one that could. The two groups were followed over time. He compared their grades, SAT scores, achievements in school, social competence, delinquency rates, and personal effectiveness (self-reliance, confidence, trustworthiness, and dependability). The group choosing to delay gratification had more positive outcomes each year on all measures (Mischel & Peake, 1990).

This is what the philosophers in chapter 1 talked about when they pitted reason against emotion. Here, we have the key piece of the development of judgment. Can we put our wants on hold long enough to consider what best would serve our long-term needs? This does not mean we must deny what we want or repress our emotions. It simply means bringing intelligence into our emotional decisions. In the long run, the 4-year-olds who delayed gratification doubled the satiation of their desire for marshmallows.

This pitting of reason against emotion is an essential skill in daily living. It is helpful in friendships, career, saving for retirement, love, and relationships. It is what is meant by self-mastery or self-control. It is one of the most important elements in what we call maturity.

ADD or ADHD and the Brain

Both children and adults have difficulty focusing interest. We know what we are supposed to be paying attention to, but we cannot seem to keep our focus on task. Many times the problem is in the way we are wired. Something is wrong with the ascending reticular activating system (ARAS). Remember, this is the system that filters out stimuli that are irrelevant to our purpose (Lindsley, 1957). When it is not working, it is difficult to control our attention and our impulses.

This is one of the few areas in which I suggest taking medications. When there is something amiss with the arousal system in the brain, stimulating that system with the right medication gives the arousal system a boost and helps us begin to control our focus.

Using this theory, the same thing can be done by a teacher in class with a girl whose mind tends to wander. The teacher can boost her arousal system by stimulating her startle response, much like Robin Williams did as he played a teacher in the movie *The Dead Poets Society*. He unexpectedly jumped up on his desk and shouted, "Carpe diem." The teacher can come up behind a student without warning and shout her name. This might well jolt her out of her seat, stimulate her ARAS for a time, and help her pay better attention. But it might get the teacher in trouble, as it did Robin Williams.

Low levels of serotonin are associated with poor impulse control (Buck, 1988). This is why physicians often combine prescriptions of Ritalin with Zoloft. Individuals who need this medication quickly report its effects. Sometimes these patients like how it helps them gain self-control, and sometimes they resent the way that it inhibits the flow of energy in their brains.

ADD, ADHD, and Partners and Parents

Often individuals with Attention Deficit Disorder (ADD) are brilliant and charming. For these reasons, we are attracted to partnering with them. In other cases, we love them because they are our children. Individuals who cannot focus need a system to filter information and to help them focus on the next step. These are the systems taught by the therapists who treat ADD and Attention Deficit Hyperactivity Disorder (ADHD).

The job of the partner or parent is to create an environment of organization around people who have difficulty focusing their attention. Examples of such a structure might include lists, places to put things, habit-building around routine. The partner or parent should keep routines simple and avoid overstimulation. Rooms should not have an abundance of color or objects. Sometimes, individuals who cannot focus should just sit for a time in the dark. This calms and rests people overwhelmed with energy and stimuli and helps them regain their emotional balance.

Easily overstimulated individuals often resist organized systems—the drugs and the lists. Have you ever seen a child want to go to bed or be glad when a parent suggests, "It's bedtime." It is rare. This is the resistance those who suffer from attention deficit must battle constantly.

Sometimes we can associate this impulsivity with addiction. People with ADD sometimes use alcohol or drugs or adrenaline (in the case of gambling, shopping, and work addicts) to calm their impulsivity. Treating addiction effectively often comes only after someone confesses to the therapist, "I've hit bottom. I need help, and I will do whatever it takes." Needless to say, we more easily can treat ADD persons who are not addicts and who have this attitude.

Bipolar Disorder

The same brain deficits that were previously described for ADD and ADHD apply to the person with bipolar disorder. Often children progress diagnostically from ADD to ADHD to Oppositional Defiant Disorder (ODD) to bipolar disorder. The good news is that bipolar disorder is treatable. The bad news is that even with treatment, this is a difficult problem to manage. Clients often prefer how they feel when they are not on the medication. But the rest of us may suffer when they refuse treatment.

Frequently, these clients are accused of addiction to adrenaline, and they will create chaos just to get another dose. Domestic violence can be part of this illness, and such individuals are often in trouble with the law.

In my 28 years of practice, only one client suffering from a bipolar disorder has asked to take the medication. Many have refused to take the medication that sometimes helps.

Psychiatrist colleagues of mine have confirmed my experience with bipolar disorder. Drugs only "sometimes" help. Usually this medication is a combination of lithium or depacote, with an SSRI (Selective Serotonin Reuptake Inhibitor) anti-depressant that increases the level of serotonin in the body. These SSRI's seem to work for a time, and then they cease to be effective. Often switching to a different SSRI is helpful.

All in all, finding the right medication is sometimes difficult, and the positive effect of the discovery can be temporary.

The Purpose of Life

If desire is stupid, as I said earlier, and, when we get what we want, we are still unhappy, then what is the point?

The point is that wanting means we are alive. Wanting keeps us moving. Without desire, we would never accomplish anything. What if we were happy when we got what we wanted? That feels rather smug, doesn't it? Perhaps it is a good thing for ourselves and the species that we keep on discovering new desires after successes and after failures. Because we are programmed this way, striving, growing, learning, and becoming are always a part of our lives from birth until death. Would you have it any other way? This is what makes life a process and makes the destination silly.

Resolving Interest/Desire/Excitement

There are two questions here. The first is: How do we resolve an interest that becomes so focused that it becomes an obsession or addiction? The second is: How do we resolve interest when we cannot seem to focus on an object or task? How do we manage a mind that races out of control?

Many times these problems are one in the same. That is why the answers to both questions are similar. They are the same, because the people who seemingly cannot focus their attention gravitate to an interest or drug strong enough to hold their interest. Often ADD and bipolar sufferers become alcoholics, because they feel that "something is not right up there" and they are searching for the drug that will fix it or at least turn it off.

To the first question: How to resolve addiction? Addiction cannot be treated until or unless we are sad, so sad that we cannot continue in the state of addiction. Some clients are suicidal at this point. It must be clear to them that their life, as they have lived it, must change. Often they are so ashamed of what they have done that they can barely face reality. They are afraid that they will only keep their addiction. This feeling of sadness, fear, and shame is the bottom. At this point, these emotions can be the beginning of a healthy emotional resolution to uncontrollable desire.

When clients confess that they need help—that they cannot go on like this anymore, that they will do whatever it takes, including submitting to the authority of a specific program—the treatment for addiction can begin. Sadness and grief bring with them wisdom; fear creates arousal and stimulates the brain. Shame, as we shall see in chapter 10, is the path to honor and signals the reweaving of our social fabric.

Thom Rutledge and I developed a four-step ritual that uses this theory to help treat addiction. I use **PRIDE** as an acronym. It is as follows:

 Step 1: Point to the voice inside you that tells you to use your addiction. Name it. Then disobey that voice.

 Step 2: Receive and experience the feelings of shame beneath your desire or compulsion to surrender to your addiction. Choose one of these words that might best express your feelings:

Unimportant	Rejected
Disregarded	Powerless
Devalued	Unlovable
Accused	Unfit for Human Contact

After you have identified your feeling(s) below your compulsion, experience that feeling for twenty seconds. If you made a mistake, face it. Learn and grow from it. Let the pain teach you. Don't be afraid to feel bad for a time.

 Step 3: Identify and correct your self-perception and your behavior. You may feel unimportant, disregarded, and so forth, but remind yourself that you are not. A mistake does not define your soul. You have had the courage to feel your pain and learn from it. This makes you important, worthy of regard and respect, valuable, never to blame for everything, never rejected by yourself, never powerless as long as you can control your feelings, always lovable, and always deserving of human compassion and contact. Tell yourself the truth about your worth, and, if you need to change your behavior and make amends, start working on that now. Do what you believe is the next right thing.

 Step 4: Detect the pride that comes from doing what's right. As you have reminded yourself that you are worthy, valuable, important, powerful, and lovable, and as you have done your best to do the right thing, feel the pride and honor that is a natural consequence of believing in yourself and doing what you believe is right. You have just had the courage to disobey your addiction voice, feel painful feelings, put these feelings in perspective, and do the right thing. You have a right to feel pride in this victory over your addiction.

 Step 5. Engage life with self-respect. "Get out among 'em." Take considered risks. Be a part of humankind without your addiction.

The second question has to do with controlling a mind that races and cannot seem to focus. Of course, *fear* will resolve interest. Fear works well, because it provides a stimulant and helps the mind focus on the object of fear. But fear also creates a mind that races to find a way out of danger, one that is confused with doubt. In the end, fear usually only adds to the problem.

Anger works most effectively. It focuses the brain and filters out external stimuli and thoughts. The problem with anger is that it is stupid, and it gives us permission to follow aggressive impulses that are poorly considered. When we search for a way to focus our minds and when we settle on anger as our choice, we usually get into more trouble.

Sadness is a better choice for building a healthy resolve for out-of-control interest. Sadness brings with it judgment and our best sense, but sadness has no arousal component. We need arousal to sharpen our focus. *Surprise/ startle/wonder* stimulates the arousal system, but its purpose is to inquire and ask questions. It can bring more confusion and little clarity. *Disgust* arouses. It focuses. It is especially useful if it can concentrate on a behavior that can become self-defeating (for example, gambling, promiscuous sex, overeating). The problem with disgust is that we can easily become the object of our own disgust.

Joy would be a great resolve to interest. In fact, joy is the natural resolve to a desire. It is how we feel after we achieve what we desire. The problem here is that our interest cannot keep a focus long enough to achieve a goal. *Sleep/rest/relaxation/trance* is perhaps the best natural drug we can give ourselves. Reducing our level of stimulation, turning down the activity in our heads, letting go, and being still can help us rebalance and clear our minds. Then, we can begin again, renewed and refreshed, filtering out unnecessary stimuli, and letting our interest rise naturally and more slowly from rest. The CALMS technique described in chapter 6 on fear might be a helpful resolution to our unfocused energy.

Resolving Craig's Problem with Interest/Desire/Excitement

I haven't emphasized enough that we all need help when our interest problems get out of control. When our desire becomes an obsession, few of us can move toward a healthy relationship with ourselves or others without compassionate help from friends. Sometimes we get in a trap like Craig and cannot get out by ourselves. In my practice, I have never seen a man involved in a love triangle who could resolve his problem alone. Usually, one or both of his lovers eventually become exhausted and leave. Craig needed help and came to me. Craig pleaded, "I will do whatever it takes. Please help me. I can no longer trust myself."

"I will help you," I said, "but I'm not sure you will like my prescription."

"I've got to take somebody's medicine," he conceded. "It might as well be yours."

"The truth is my medicine," I said. "I think your wife deserves the truth. And then, if she wants to help you, I think she can help put solid boundaries around your marriage so that you can work together to rebuild your relationship. If she wants out, she has the truth, and she can use it to leave now. That would resolve this dilemma. Craig, I don't think you are strong enough to do this yourself. I think you need her help."

Craig invited his wife Enid to the next session in which he told her about Lindsay. "There . . . now I'm sure you want a divorce," Craig said, as he ended his confession.

"No, Craig, I don't," Enid replied. "I've been married to you for 23 years. I am 47. My youth and beauty are gone. A divorce from you now would leave me broke, old, and fat."

"You're not old or fat," Craig countered.

"You have not an idea," Enid answered. "You are not going to go out on the market. Lindsay is rich, younger than I am, and very pretty. She will have no trouble finding a new husband, if that's what she wants. I have 23-years-plus courtship years invested in you, in us, Craig. I'm not about to throw them away. I'm mad as hell at you, but I'm going to fight for my marriage. I can't stop you from leaving me and getting a divorce. But if you want to work on us, that's what I want to do, too. Is that what you want to do?"

"Yes, I think so."

"Is that the best you can do? 'I think so.' Damn you, Craig."

"That is the best he can do," I said. "He is confused and lost. If your marriage is to be protected from this threat, you need to protect it. Craig is too weak to do it."

"How can I do it?" she asked.

"Lindsay sees you as a disembodied obstacle, a competitor," I said, "and you see her as an interloper or worse."

"That's right, worse," she said.

"Well, Lindsay didn't break her marriage vows," I said. "Lindsay had no professional responsibility not to prey on clients when needy herself. All Lindsay did was find this man attractive and respond to that attraction, just as you once did. You both have similar taste in men. I suspect you have a great deal in common."

"Yeah, Lindsay looks like I did 10 years ago," Enid said. "Same color hair, about my size, same haircut. My hair is white now and short, and my middle is not flat anymore."

"Cut it out about how you look, Enid," Craig said. "You look fine to me."

"If that's true then . . ."

I interrupted. "Back to protecting your marriage. Enid, you need to meet with Lindsay and tell her what you told Craig today, that you mean to keep your marriage. It would be easy to make her the villain, but she's not. Craig betrayed you; she didn't. Craig needs to resolve this by being sad, ashamed, making amends, and rediscovering joy with you. Once it is safe, you, Enid, need to understand your contribution to what went wrong. Craig will never get past his grief, make amends with you, and reestablish himself as your equal partner as long as you remain the righteous, innocent victim and Craig the only sinner. If this marriage is to work, both of you must be confessional to the other. Ask the question sincerely, 'What would it be like to be married to me?'"

"I've been asking myself that question lately," Enid said. "And I didn't like the answer that came to me. Craig is in this spot because of my greed. We have a nice house. Craig makes a good living. I don't need to be a queen in my palace. I put too much pressure on Craig to build my dream house. That was my fault. I couldn't forgive him. I pushed him away . . ."

I interrupted again. "That's good, but that work we can do later. Right now you have to reestablish your boundaries. Craig, if you want this marriage to work, you must end your relationship with Lindsay. Your loyalty must be to Enid. Can you do that?"

"I don't know," he said. "Right here, that's what I think I should do. I want to want that. I do want that at some level, but maybe I can't. When I heard you, Enid, take some of the blame for this mess, that felt good. I feel so guilty all the time. You have no idea."

"I can help you with that," Enid said. "But I'm not sure I can help you with Lindsay."

"Oh, yes, you can," I said. "Affairs only can exist in secret. Once Lindsay and you are sharing information, the affair or the marriage will end."

"It won't be the marriage, if I can help it," Enid said.

Craig's work to resolve this "wanting too much" is to relearn delay of gratification, grieve, let go, feel sad about what was lost, refocus his interest on Enid, and follow his new goal, for example, sharing joy with Enid. Luckily, their children provided them with a source of shared pride. Once their relationship boundaries were established, their task was to spend time together, protecting each other from shame, being proud of getting up after they fell down. From time to time, that's something all of us must do.

In the next chapter we follow the story of Enid and Craig. A second version of the PRIDE ritual is introduced there. They are nearly identical, but one is oriented toward addiction, and the second is aimed at resolving shame.

CHAPTER 10

Shame/Guilt[10]
The Most Instructive Emotion

Shame Defined

Shame is not one of Ekman's seven, but Tomkins and Izard include it on their lists. For Ekman and other emotion researchers, shame is a combination of fear and sadness. For them, it is not a basic emotion. It is number one among most therapists as the cause of psychopathology (Nathanson, 1992).

While shame does not emerge in the infant for some time after birth, I contend that it is a basic emotion. Perhaps infant brains require some experience in a relationship before the brain can mature enough to experience shame. Just because it is not present at birth does not mean it is not a singular affect.

If shame were a constellation of fear and sadness, shame would likely be an avoidance emotion. Fear is an avoidant emotion and sadness is an emotion that has neither an approach or avoid valence. A combination of the two would encourage withdrawal.

Though we all have an impulse to withdraw from the pain of shameful circumstances, shame serves the social function of healing relationships. In this sense, shame is an approach emotion. It connotes submission and a seeking of forgiveness. It is an invitation to reconnect on the basis of a reconfiguration of the power structure. In dogs, it is an approach with tail between the hind legs. In monkeys, it is a coy, embarrassed, shy, contrite approach.

Most of us hate to feel shame, and we do a poor job of processing or transforming it into something healthy. We all know what shame is. It is often called a "loss of face," which means a de-elevation of our public respect and reputation, a fall from grace. It is a sudden realization that we have done wrong, torn the fabric of trust we once had with a friend. When we feel shame, our neck turns red; our head turns down and away from the person that we believe was wronged.

Shame is painful. It stops pleasure in its tracks and reins in whatever action we were taking. Our thoughts suddenly become confused, and we behave awkwardly and submissively toward the person whom we now feel has good reason to disapprove of us.

Many theorists distinguish between shame and guilt (Lewis, 1971; Kugler & Jones, 1992). Some say we feel guilt over what we did and shame over who we are. For our purposes here, guilt and shame are the same. They look the same on the face, and they feel the same in the body. Some other words that are represented in this emotion are humiliation, embarrassment, and mortification.

Tomkins (1963) said that "shame is the affect of indignity of transgression and of alienation....Shame strikes the deepest in the heart of man. Shame is felt as an inner torment, a sickness of the soul. It does not matter whether the humiliated one has been

shamed by derisive laughter, or whether he mocks himself. In either one, he feels himself naked, defeated, alienated, and lacking in dignity or worth" (p. 118).

Shame can be a socialization tool. Shame becomes an important source of social bonding. It motivates us to accept our share of the responsibility for the good of the whole (Izard, 1971; Lewis, 1971; Tomkins, 1962).

Shame focuses on and exposes our weaknesses and inadequacies. It exposes our sense of ineptness. It directs our attention to work we need to do to strengthen our skills and heal our relationships (Tomkins, 1963; Lewis, 1971; Tangney, Miller, Flicker, & Barlos, 1996; Izard, 1971).

When we feel ashamed, we sense that we have done something wrong and that we will submit and accept the consequences. Healthy shame is a measure of our bonds to others and of our concern and sense of responsibility for their well-being. When we are unable to accept responsibility and pay the consequences for our behavior that harms others, shame can grow into a deep, unhealthy feeling that is toxic to our sense of self.

Clinical Case Study

I continued my work with Craig and referred Enid to another therapist. I also worked with Enid and Craig as a couple, and sometimes we would meet conjointly with the second therapist. But here, I am reporting a session with Craig. Enid had successfully met with Lindsay. Lindsay bowed out gracefully and was soon enjoying being single, rich, and attractive. But Craig felt stuck.

"Before it was wanting that I hated. Now it is shame," he explained. I can't seem to get past the guilt I feel. I was mostly sad at first. But as soon as I heard about Lindsay dating and saw her picture with other men in the society pages, I realized that she was better off and so was I. Enid was great. She met with Lindsay. She did such a good job that I didn't even have to call Lindsay. Lindsay called me and said our affair was over.

"It was a good feeling to know that Enid cared that much. But I still couldn't look at Enid and feel anything but guilt. I had been guilty over losing our money and her dream home. Added to that, I felt guilt over betraying her with Lindsay. I had always prided myself in being honest. My integrity was my most important asset. I lied and cheated in ways I didn't know I was capable of. I not only broke my marriage vows, but I began to lie to my colleagues, my secretary. I got to the place where I didn't know who I was or what I was going to do next.

"I'm glad that I am out of that sleazy, deceptive life. But now I am having a hard time living with what I did. I still can't believe it was me. But it was me. My job is to be able to get past guilt when I see Enid. I know she has a great sense of humor. She is a wonderful lover. She has even propositioned me a couple of times. But I can't seem to get through my shame to my desire.

"Love and guilt don't mix. How can I look at Enid without guilt, if I can't look at myself in the mirror?"

The Neurology of Shame

According to Nathanson (1992), shame is the most highly evolved emotion. It depends on the others for its existence. Shame interferes with positive affect and mobilizes the pain of sadness and fear. He conjectures that shame secretes an as yet undiscovered neurochemical into the subcortical portion of the brain that somehow causes the dilation of the brain's blood vessels and arteries. Shame causes the eyes to drop and the head to droop. Sometimes, in a moment of shame, our whole body wilts and becomes confused.

Any description of how shame works in the brain is speculation on my part. I would suggest that shame has to do with the submission half of the dominance/ submission response, the punishment half of the punishment/ reward system, as well as having a link to depression and fear and the play and nurture/affection part of the brain.

The submission part of the dominance/submission reflex is located primarily in the hypothalamus. The anterior region of the hypothalamus is associated with submission behaviors. The punishment part of the reward/ punishment system is associated with the periventricular system (PVS) (Olds & Olds, 1963).

When shame acts to separate us from loved ones, the distress we feel is registered in the anterior and preoptic area (POA) of the hypothalamus (Panksepp, 1982). In the limbic system, the cingulate cortex is also associated with the separation distress cry (Scott, 1974).

De Wall and Aureli (1997) speculated that these areas of the brain are active in chimpanzees when they feel they have done wrong. Reconciliation appears to be species-determined behavior in chimpanzees following intra-species fighting. After fighting, the behaviors of hugging, kissing, grooming, and making-up follow. Nearby chimpanzees often offer consolation to the submitting loser. The left hemisphere of the brain appears to be particularly associated with shame.

In a recent article, Shin, Dougherty, Orr, Pittman, Lasko, Macklin, Alport, Fischman, and Rauch (2000) became the first researchers to map the neuro-anatomy of shame. They found that shame activated the anterior paralimbic structures of the brain, specifically the anterior cingulate gyrus, the left anterior insular cortex of the inferior frontal gyrus, and the bilateral anterior temporal poles. This finding is consistent with one associating the anterior paralimbic regions of the brain with negative emotions, such as sadness and fear (Derryberry & Tucker, 1992).

Buck (1999) tells the story of a woman whose brain was being operated on. Before the operation, she said that she was angry at people who teased her about her epilepsy as a child. When the left hemisphere was deactivated with a dose of sodium ambitrol, she stated that she was embarrassed and ashamed by the abuse, rather than angry.

A man receiving similar treatment reported that he was angry and frustrated at physicians who couldn't diagnose his illness properly. Once his left hemisphere had been rendered inactive, he said that he felt "sorry for people that had so much trouble finding out what was wrong."

These stories suggest the importance of the left hemisphere to shame.

We can identify several neurohormone candidates that induce shame. High levels of monoamine oxidase (MAO) are associated with introversion and withdrawal (Buck, 1999). The pain peptide neurotransmitter substance P is likely to have high levels associated with shame, as well as the fear neurohormone choleceptotonin (CCK), which increases blood flow to the limbic area (MacLean, 1993).

I described in chapter 6 on fear how the corticotrophin-releasing hormone (CRF) depleted the brain of its ability to balance itself. High levels of CRF coordinate our body's central stress response (Panksepp 1993). The action of this hormone explains how guilt about a failure in one event, or series of events, can be transformed into shame as a state, shame of the self. Norepinephrine (NA) inhibits this fear/anxiety stress hormone (CRF), and CRF in turn excites norepinephrine. If CRF continues to be released, it exhausts the supply of its antagonist, norepinephrine.

What we have left is a chronic state of despair and perhaps self-hatred and shame, because our brain has no CRF antagonists to reduce CRF levels in the brain (Risch, 1991).

Low levels of the endorphins that induce pleasure and reduce pain are likely associated with shame. High levels of serotonin (5-H7) are associated with dominance and ego strength. Low levels of serotonin, therefore, likely would be associated with shame, as well as low levels of the gonadotropin-releasing hormone (GnRH) for the same reasons. "Oxytocin is a prime candidate for mediating feelings of social acceptance," (Pankseep, 1993, p. 93). Consequently, shame is likely to suppress it, as well as vasopressin (VP), which is associated with intraspecies and sexual aggression.

Most of this is speculation, with the exception of the Shin study (Shin, et al., 2000). Neurological research on the experience of shame in the brain has been impeded, because shame has not been considered a basic or natural emotion. More research needs to be done so that speculations, such as those offered here, can be confirmed or refuted and accurate data can take their place.

Physiology and Shame

The dilation of the blood vessels exhibited by blushing is the most obvious physical marker of shame, together with the drooping face that looks away (Nathanson, 1992). So little research exists on the anatomy of shame that we are reduced to speculation about how the body reacts to shame.

Again, a reason for this is that shame is not considered a primary emotion but rather a derivative one. I would speculate that when we feel shame, our blood pressure lowers, our heart rate slows, and our general muscle tone and arousal drops.

Perhaps researchers soon will give us more information about the physiology of shame.

The Intelligence of Shame

Using research conducted by Shin and others, we can begin to speculate on whether shame fills our brain with confusion, as Nathanson suggested, or whether shame is connected to the neocortex, bringing with it major problem-solving capacities (Shin, et al., 2000). Shin's study suggests an extensive neural network similar to that related to sadness.

If the function of shame is to reveal to us the work we need to do to improve ourselves and our skills, it makes sense that shame brings with it some formidable intellectual capacity. I believe that after the initial shock and exposure of shame, the whole brain gets to work, trying to figure out how what happened wasn't really our fault. Once we have finished trying to shift the blame, shame motivates us to learn how to avoid more shame by facing the task of self-improvement, so as not to make the same mistake again.

The Negative Consequences of Shame

Guilt/shame is an emotion that we try to avoid. The reason for this is that shame hurts. It hurts to admit to being wrong. It hurts to take responsibility for our behavior. It is often in running away from shame that the worst of the pathology from shame occurs. We often perform extraordinary mental gymnastics to push guilt away from us and onto others, because we lack the courage to look at our own harmful behavior and accept responsibility.

On the other hand, we can feel too much shame. When this happens, we believe that the core of our essential self is shameful and that we are unfit for human contact.

Guilt, like anger, fear, and sadness, has an unhealthy face. It is healthy when we accept guilt for harmful behavior or a mistake that hurts someone else. It is not healthy when we believe we and our mistakes are one in the same.

The purpose of shame is to close down behavior so that we cannot continue on a potentially destructive path. The socially constructive function of shame is to mend a social fabric that has been torn. Shame used correctly rebuilds, reconnects, and reties. When shame becomes pathological, we can care too much about righting the wrongs that cannot be righted or pleasing people who cannot be pleased or who become tyrants empowered by our shame. When this happens, instead of feeling empowered and reconnected by processing shame, we become stuck in shame. We feel closed down, dead to ourselves, choked, confined, imprisoned, too close, too exposed, needing distance, more clothes, or other defenses—somewhat like being on stage and required to perform when we don't know our lines. This "I-want-to-crawl-under-a-rock-and-hide" feeling is painful. In circumstances that require us to sacrifice our dignity and well-being for peace, shame becomes what Thom Rutledge (2002) calls a "should monster." Instead of redeeming and enabling, shame punishes and becomes a resource for evil.

The toxicity of extreme shame—the way it makes us feel shameful to our core—is the psychological engine of compulsive-addictive behavior. Some of us use consumption of food, drugs, sex, excitement, for example, as a drug to rescue us from guilt. This kind of consumption focuses our attention on an addictive experience that is intense enough to displace guilt and pleasurable enough to shift our emotional focus.

Compulsive behavior is any behavior we repeat that common sense tells us is unnecessary or not good for us but that we don't seem to be able to stop ourselves from doing. Compulsive behavior leads to more shame, because we know we shouldn't do what we are doing. This guilt leads to more compulsive behavior, and the toxic shame cycle continues.

How does unhealthy shame develop? Parents and teachers might promote toxic shame in children by mishandling the emotion of guilt. Mishandling guilt can be a matter of ignoring opportunities for teaching children useful lessons about guilt. As authorities to children, we miss these chances when we don't correct children for behavior that hurts others. For example, we hurt the child when we ignore his saying mean things, when he excludes others in an unkind way, or is violent with others. These narcissistic errors need to be learned from. The child needs his consciousness raised to appreciate the feelings of others. Opportunities for this learning should not be missed.

Mishandling guilt can also be a matter of inflicting penalties that are inherently shaming to the child/offender, for example, hitting the child or verbally abusing her. We now criticize parents who spank children, once a fairly common disciplinary measure, because parents often strike in anger, giving the child the message that she deserves physical cruelty enacted in rage. If, as children, we were frequently punished with spanking, we probably felt overpowered, angry, shamed, afraid, but seldom contrite. Penalties are effective in teaching us to feel a healthy guilt when we also have the ego-strength to make amends for the harm we have caused, but not when these penalties strip us of our dignity and make us feel powerless and unworthy.

If clients do not learn how to manage guilt in a healthy way—if they do not learn how to confess, apologize, make amends, rebuild trust—they likely will continue to avoid this painful emotion. Avoiding guilt, however, usually does not eliminate it. When we are afraid of guilt, we begin to work hard, instead, to hide our secret sense of shame. We feel more guilty because of this, not less.

In addition to mishandling guilt, we also might try to pass on our own shame to others, especially our children. Parents who can't manage their own guilt might, for example, call their children names (e.g., guilty mother to a child who wants more time for herself: "Can't you see I'm busy. You're so selfish!") or blame them for conditions that the children cannot control (e.g., guilty father to a child whose mother needs more help from the father: "Your mother never got mad until you were born! Now she is angry all the time.").

Teaching your clients about guilt has two components. First, you must teach them how to make guilt a manageable emotion, one that has its proper place in character development and is part of a client's developing a capacity to love. Second, you must work to inoculate your client and yourself against toxic shame.

The Positive Consequences of Shame

Because guilt/shame is such a difficult emotion to endure, we often do not see its benefits immediately. Guilt/shame is an important part of the attachment bond or what most of us call love. If we have the courage to love others, we accept responsibility for being a source of good for them. If, instead, we are a source of ill, our love makes us feel guilty.

This is the healthy face of guilt. The guilt I feel for doing harm to you is a sign that I love you. It signals that I have broken a loving bond, and guilt helps me rebuild a secure, safe human attachment. It is the primary feeling that supports social responsibility. Although guilt is painful and you might wish to spare your client painful experiences, remember this healthy link between love and guilt. If your client is not willing or able to feel guilt, she also lacks the capacity to love.

Character lessons are those often painful lessons that we must learn in order to develop into mature human beings. We recognize that we have had a character lesson when we struggle with shame. As we work to come to grips with this emotion, we often recognize a truth about ourselves, one that we might have been unaware of or even tried to deny.

The primary character lessons we learn in our lives often are a product of the guilt we feel, because we have made a mistake that has hurt someone we care about. In this way, guilt is our teacher and builds our character.

Making Shame Healthy

For some of us, shame does not come and then go. For some of us, shame is a constant emotional state. It is a cloud that follows us everywhere. This cloud can become a belief that at the base of our identity we are poison. We come to believe that there is something wrong in us that we cannot fix, and we are afraid others will find that out.

This belief is a lie. None of us is perfect. All of us have personality flaws, but these flaws are not the whole of who we are. Consider our bodies. About 2% of our physical bodies is poison. Our urine and feces contain bacteria and waste that is disgusting. But this 2% is not the whole of us. We have parts of our bodies that we are grateful for, feet that walk, arms that hold, ears that hear, eyes that see. Sometimes we forget about the blessings we have to share with the world and focus only on the parts of ourselves that we wish to reject.

Though none of us enjoys guilt, we can get beyond it. If we identify shame as the base of our personal pain, we must tell the truth about who we are. Remember, a mistake is just a mistake; we can make amends for it, correct it or learn from it, and go forward and see the good in our whole selves.

Our clients can understand and appreciate guilt only if they see their mistakes as mistaken behavior and not as an indication of essential flaws in the core of their beings. When they believe that the guilt comes from something wrong with their soul, they rightly will reject the guilt and lose the opportunity to learn the lesson it has to teach them.

Clients look to us as their therapists to see what we reflect to them in our eyes. If they see disgust and contempt reflected in our expression, they will feel that way about themselves. They will not feel empowered to make amends for their mistakes. They will not feel that guilt is a starting place where they can ask how to repair the harm they have done. Instead, they will feel rejected, possibly angry for a while, and very likely hopeless about themselves. They might withdraw into the belief that they are evil and give up trying to be socially acceptable.

Just as shame is an essential part of the human glue we call love, it also nurtures us, providing the milk of human kindness. In the film *Notting Hill*, with Hugh Grant and Julia Roberts, the writers created a scene early in the movie in which Grant collides with Roberts and spills orange juice on her. He is ashamed and guilty. He apologizes and tries his best to right the wrong. Immediately, the audience identifies with him as a kind, sympathetic character, because he is so ashamed and tries so hard to make amends.

Being kind means that when things go wrong, we give the other person the benefit of the doubt, point the finger of blame at ourselves, and say, "Oh, my goodness, what did I do to create this mess?! I'm sorry. Here, let me help." This shame statement is the essence of kindness.

Shame is such a simple emotion, one that is useful every day. On the face of it, shame seems so easy. All it is: "Oops, I'm sorry. I made a mistake. I feel bad about that. I won't do that again." All of us are in a position to make this simple confession several times a day. Many of us have difficulty finding these words.

The reason shame is difficult to confess is not just because we hate being wrong or facing a mistake. It is not just because of the painful feeling that comes with shame. The primary reason that shame is so difficult is that shame requires us to learn, grow, and change. An "I'm-sorry" means nothing without commitment to behave differently, and the commitment means nothing without change. Shame means that we cannot afford to sit back and accept ourselves as we are; the status quo is not acceptable. Shame is a confession that we are not there yet. We have work to do, consciousness to raise, new and better behaviors to learn. Most of us would rather believe that we are fine just the way we are. We don't want to take on the challenges that shame requires.

Learning to use the daily challenge shame gives us to grow is an important lesson. Knowing how to use shame means that we are strong enough to bear the burdens of living with people we love. It says that we can be a good friend, partner, or lover. Shame used this way is something that we can be proud to feel. This is something that we all want to learn and pass on to our children.

Shame used this way is simply the process of facing a mistake. We make many mistakes in our everyday existence. Shame in this context comes with a confession and goes away with making amends. This is an important lesson for us and for our clients to pass on to our children as well.

A 4-year-old has a difficult time with shame. Not until a child is 6, 7, or 8 years old, can she begin to use shame effectively (Ferguson, Stegge, Miller, & Olson, 1999). The capacity to use shame as a part of daily living comes simultaneously with our ability to express compassion.

Young children should not be directly challenged to engage shame. But parents can do certain things to prepare their children for the time when they will be able to use shame effectively. Children look at their parents to see how they should treat their mistakes. If their parents react to their children's mistakes passionately or violently with anger and disgust, their children will have great difficulty developing a healthy relationship with shame. If parents treat their children's mistakes as things that happen that can be fixed, events that we know they did not intend to create; if they meet their parents' expectations to right the wrong and make the amends, the parents have taught their children how to take the right path with shame. Parents should be proud of their children for this and proud of themselves as teachers.

It is important that you remind your clients of their strengths. Shame is the emotional cutting edge of learning and growing. Remind your clients that they don't need to be afraid of the change that is part of amends-making because they can change. They are always changing. If a child's small hand dropped a glass of milk, you would remind her to use two hands, of course, but also remind her that her hands are growing. Holding a glass will become easier. Shouldn't we do the same for our clients?

If a child made a mistake cutting out a figure, we would remind her that with practice she will get better using scissors. Shouldn't we do this for our clients, too—help them remember that they have many strengths and talents? Part of a therapist's job is to keep reminding clients about their strengths. Remind them they can apply their talents to the learning, growing, and the changing that we all must do when we make a mistake and feel bad. It is just a mistake. With their ability to grow and learn, they can make the needed change to mend their relationships with others. All this change requires is caring and paying attention; the subsequent growth and change will come with practice and time, and the memory of the pain that came from their shame will fade.

Your job with your clients is to keep in front of them their talents, strengths, and capacities for growing. Our development is not static. Change will come. With your clients' considerable, unique skills, they can direct their talents so that they become better at whatever it is they want to accomplish.

You must succeed in helping your clients learn to use shame effectively so that they do not become defined by shame. Shame is a tool, not a constant way to feel. Without experiencing the emotional lessons inherent in shame, no other emotional lessons can be learned.

Knowing What to Expect of Ourselves

Many emotional responses to stimuli have to do with expectations. Joy, for example, can come when our expectations are exceeded. Shame can come when we fail to meet our expectations. Shame is especially painful if others shared our expectations and were depending on us to meet them—and we did not.

As a sophomore in high school, when I played on my high school golf team, I was usually third or fourth man, depending on the outcome of the prematch qualifying round. Ed McCorkle was usually second. On this particular qualifying day, I was playing well. On the 8th hole, I got confused about my score for that hole. It was a par 5. Ed had a 7 on that hole. As I counted my score, I had a 6. But I wasn't sure whether or not I omitted one shot. Rather than being sure of my score, I blurted out that I had a 6. The coach challenged me, but I was committed to my 6 by this time, and I repeated that I had a 6. As a result, I became second man on our golf team for the first time.

On the day of the match, I tried to pump myself up. I bragged that I was going to beat my opponent and that the number one and two men, as a team, would win our match. Our coach shook his head. "David," he said, "you are cruising for a bruising." And he was right. I shot an 87. I lost. The first-and-second-man team lost. Our team, as a whole, lost. If I had played third man, my usual position, I would have tied my opponent. Ed shot an 82. His score, with the first man's score, would have won the match for us.

I was ashamed of my conduct and my play. I tried to be more than I was. The other members of my team have probably forgotten that match. But I haven't, and I don't think I ever will. Perhaps the pain of my shame and this memory was worth it. I did learn a lesson about staying within the limits of my ability and how important it is to keep my score correctly. But I still feel the pain of this character error, as I write this.

We often watch our clients as they set themselves up for failure, as I did by trying to be the second man when I was really the third. We must not contribute to this by seeing strengths in our clients that they do not possess. We must value them for who they are, respect them for the quality of their effort and for their courage when they take risks. We should care less about outcomes and more about our clients' willingness to try, helping keep them in life's game, putting out effort, learning from mistakes, and trying again.

That is life at its best. And it is our job to help clients focus on the journey and not on the destination (Buddha's grandfather, 500 B.C.).

Center of the Universe or Star-Player Defense

Children often believe that the world revolves around them, that they are the center of the universe. Whatever happens is because of them. If their favorite team wins, it was because they were watching every at-bat on television. If their parents get a divorce, it is because they were bad and their parents were fighting over how and whether their child should be punished.

I have come to believe that psychological maturity followed the same evolutionary principle as "ontogeny recapitulates phylogeny." Although I'm still not sure, I think it means that the neonate in the womb begins looking like an amoeba, then evolves into something that looks like a tadpole, then a monkey, and then a human.

Well, I think that our psychological maturity follows the evolution of knowledge. Like the people before Copernicus who believed that the earth was the center of the universe and the sun revolved around it, the most childish of us believe that we are responsible for all that happens. As we grow up, we see how silly we were even to think that. We see how small we are and of what little consequence we are in the greater scheme of things. The wiser we become, the smaller we become.

This relates to shame, because when we believe that we are responsible for life's outcomes—involving others and ourselves—failure is inevitable. Shame will become a constant. When we see that we are a small player, just one force with the privilege to be playing in this world with others playing beside us, with us, against us, then playing becomes a privilege. The outcomes become something that fate determines together with other individuals. We have a contribution to make to the outcome, but it is a small one.

For example, consider the idea of emotions resolving emotions as a treatment plan and that theory is in the zeitgeist. If I don't write it this week, someone else will next week. It is a joy for me that I am able to tap into the spirit of Tomkins, Nathanson, Izard, and Ekman to apply, as best I can, what they taught me about how to apply emotions to clinical practice.

The extent that I believe I am essential to a task is the extent to which I will feel shame and see myself as a failure. This is a trap I often fall into.

For the benefit of our clients and ourselves, we must help them find joy in being a part of a community, rather than being the hero for the community or the victim of a community (having in their mind performed an act that should have made them the hero but didn't, because the community just didn't understand their intent).

The Joy of Accountability

The most common problem with shame is that we run away from it. We don't face shame, experience it, learn from it, and grow because of it. We blame others. We search for a way to say, "It is not my fault." When we point the finger at someone else and say, "It's your fault. You are accountable for it. You fix it," we are giving them the power to change. As long as we blame others, we remain their passive innocent victims. When we blame others, although we may escape blame, we give away our power to influence the future. Innocence and goodness have no growing or learning to do. When a teacher creates a test where all the students attain perfect scores, it means that they have nothing to learn. But if the teacher gives a test where no one gets a perfect score, the students have learned from taking the test the areas in which they are weak. They learn what they need to work on in order to master the subject.

All of us who need to grow, who are not innocent, have work to do. We need to practice more, play more. With that we will change and grow. Being at fault gives us something that we can do. That is power. Being the innocent victim, pointing and blaming others, renders us powerless. We have to wait for them to change in order for our lives to change.

To know what our work is requires that we become accountable, that we keep the correct score. Sorry, but here is another golfing story that illustrates my point.

I was playing golf with my friend, Bob Maynard. We both hit our drives in the left rough on the 12th hole, a par 5. He found what he thought was his ball, not more than 6 feet from mine. He hit his next shot. I went to what I thought was my ball and discovered that it wasn't mine, it was his. I placed my ball near where he hit his shot, and I hit my second shot. He then hit his actual ball. When we finished the hole, both of us had struck a ball 5 times. I was keeping score, and I asked for the scores from all the players. "Seven," Bob called out.

"Seven," I said. "You had a 5. I was watching."

"No," Bob said, "I had a 7."

"Your drive was 1, your second shot from the rough was 2 . . ."

"No," Bob interrupted. "It's a 2-stroke penalty for hitting the wrong ball."

"I'm not going to hold you to that," I said. "I would've hit the wrong ball if you hadn't. It was more or less the same shot. You shouldn't be penalized for that. It is as much my fault as yours. I'm not going to win the hole because of that."

"Look, David," Bob said, looking very serious, "I don't know what you are playing. But I'm, playing golf. In golf there are rules, and they are the rules for a reason. If I'm going to get better at this game, I have to take the rules seriously. I want to be penalized."

"But you lose the hole unfairly," I protested.

"I want to be held accountable," Bob said. "It is my pleasure to lose the hole following the rules of golf."

I couldn't stop thinking about what Bob said. I kept hearing him say, "It is my pleasure to lose the hole. . . . I want to be held accountable." I thought about these words. I thought about how far I was from saying them myself. I was 36 at the time. Bob was 45. I knew Bob had done a good thing, something I should aspire to. But I didn't understand it.

I'm 59 now. And I know Bob Maynard today to be the same man. I honor and respect him. I now see how it was his pleasure to be held accountable. I see that he embraced his shame, and, in so doing, he discovered honor. Confessing his mistakes was a principle that he was proud to live by.

Since that time, I have wanted to be associated with honor and integrity, first, like my mentor Bob. When I have the strength, like Bob, I take some pleasure in being held accountable.

When we continue to avoid shame, we know somewhere deep inside us that something is terribly wrong. Our self-esteem rocks between extremely inflated to very low and never rests on a realistic middle ground. We become and remain isolated, because we don't take the licks we have coming. We don't make amends. We don't change. In fact, instead of changing, we avoid blame or try not to care. We don't learn from our mistakes. We are not good friends. We cannot be trusted.

When we invite shame and make amends, the joy of accountability becomes the joy of friendship and honor.

Just the Right Amount

Shame is perhaps the most difficult of our emotions to manage. Too little creates meanness and sociopathic behavior. Too much creates self-hatred and poisonous, blaming, projective defenses. Many mental-health professionals have criticized this theory saying to me that shame was only toxic. Certainly shame is too often toxic. Good people can quickly be consumed with paralyzing shame. Immature people protect themselves from shame with anger projecting blame on others.

We need shame, but we only need enough to promote accountability, grow, and change. More than that and we become emotionally sick. We can all remember times when we took on too much shame. We can see this in others. One of the clearest examples happens in sports when an athlete makes a mistake and has a fit of anger at him or herself. This happens in every game of Little League Baseball. The job of the coach is to refocus the athlete away from the mistake and back to the reality of the next pitch. Too much shame will render the athlete impotent. All that's needed is enough shame so that the athlete will remember to practice more so that this skill area becomes a second nature competence.

Having no shame will only create arrogance and an assumed entitlement to success. Forgiveness for someone with no shame will only lead to further failure and estrangement. The task for all of us is to transform the shame into positive constructive energy. An overload of shame can make this task impossible to accomplish.

Practice and Ritual

The best way to modulate shame and to prevent the pain of shame at the core of the self is through accountability and self-discipline.

Self-discipline comes from practice and ritual. It comes from structured repetition and commitment to a goal. It comes from using shame by confessing, "I'm not as good at this as I need to be. I'm sorry about that. I will practice some more, and maybe I will get better."

When we choose and accept a discipline, we will make mistakes over and over in the context of our practice. To improve, we must confess, feel shame, and accept responsibility for our mistakes. This hurts. It takes courage to feel shame. That courage is rewarded by talent development.

This progress creates a microcosm of how healthy guilt works in life. As we grow in our discipline, we will grow in our ability to accept responsibility to say, "It's my fault," to hurt because of it, and to become more determined to pay attention, do better, and avoid that pain the next time. Shame is the ally of learning inside a discipline.

This is one of the functions of religious rituals. Daily meditation and prayer, the saying of the rosary, the chanting of mantras are repetitive activities that help us confess that we have room to grow and at the same time accept that we are worthy of love and acceptance. These activities help us use shame to regain our emotional balance. Habitual spiritual behavior grounds us in our essential goodness. Religious rituals attempt to participate and communicate with the eternal and the transcendent, even though we humans often fall short of serving these values.

When we bring our shame and guilt to an authority greater than ourselves—one who expects us to be accountable and loves and accepts us even though we make mistakes or because we make mistakes and feel contrite—our imagination sometimes surrounds us with forgiveness. This confession allows us the opportunity for cleansing and redemption. Healing growth and second chances naturally flow from these religious rituals.

Shame and Addiction

Shame combined with fear can create an addiction, a compulsive desire to run toward our addiction to, for example, alcohol, work, sex, or exercise, and avoid the pain of shame. It is important to note the powerful connection between shame and addiction. Much of what can be said here is contained in chapter 9 on interest (see the PRIDE technique as it relates to addiction).

Resolving Shame

By now, you have more than an inkling of how I think shame is resolved. Nathanson's 1992 book *Shame and Pride* suggests a resolving continuum from which each of these two emotions can resolve into the other. But before we explore the resolution of shame with joy, let's consider the other emotions as resolving candidates.

Of course, all emotions resolve each other. Any emotion will take you out of shame for a moment. But not every emotion placed next to shame will lead out of shame and into a new emotional space.

Fear, for example, will resolve our shame, but probably only to return us to shame, because we might be ashamed of being afraid. *Sadness* contains much of the pain of shame. Even if sadness resolves shame, we are still in a painful emotional hole.

Anger—now here is an emotion that can sometimes work to resolve shame. But it is often difficult to reach from shame. If we do reach anger from shame, we are likely to do something stupid out of anger and fall right back into shame.

Here is an example of how anger worked effectively. My wife, Marietta, tells of a time when she was taking a world history final. She is of German origin, and the essay question she was asked to answer was: "Why did Hitler happen in Germany?" She told me of her experience when she read that question.

"I froze," she said. "It was the only time this ever happened to me. I couldn't write. I couldn't think. I couldn't go on. I left the room. I was ashamed that I came from a German family. Then, I got mad. I got mad at myself for being caught off guard in this way. I got mad at my parents who taught me German. I got mad at the Germans for being so rigid and so easily led into wrong. I got so angry that I forgot my shame for being German, and I walked back into that test and answered that question."

Most of us, when ashamed, don't have the confidence to access anger. But when we can, anger can be of considerable help as it was to Marietta. But remember, anger is stupid. It creates cognitive distortions. And acting out of anger may create more shame.

Surprise will help jolt us out of shame for a moment. But we need an emotional place to move toward when asking the question, "What's going on." After the surprise question is answered and we know what's going on, we often will fall right back into our puddle of shame.

Interest/excitement/desire can resolve shame by distracting us for a moment toward an object of desire. But once satiated, the undercurrent of shame can return to take center stage in our minds and bodies. Our eyes will look down again. Our heads will droop, and our eyes will look away as we remember our shortcomings. This is the route to addictions. Interest/excitement/desire can become a vehicle out of shame if the object of our interest is to learn how to do better and what it takes to make amends.

Sleep/relaxation/trance can give us a reprieve from shame, by distracting us. But sometimes, during sleep, our dreams only replay our shame and our fear of shame. When we wake from sleep, shame can be the emotion that we wake to feel.

Disgust, like anger, can be helpful in resolving shame. Often shame is a product of caring too much. Shame used this way closes down feelings that we believe will not be acceptable to people we wish to please. Our unspoken mental voice speaks words like: "I have had enough," "I want to throw up," "I've had it." These words imply that we are disgusted. We have eaten enough of what someone is feeding us. Shame can block us from speaking out and saying, "No," when that is exactly what we need to say. In these circumstances, disgust is an excellent resolve to shame. But as with anger, once ashamed, we are rarely in a powerful enough position to entertain disgust. And disgust, like anger, uses categorical thinking. Thinking in boxes often can lead us into serious mistakes and back to shame.

This leaves *joy*. Pride is a form of joy. Few would intuitively expect that the healthy emotional route out of shame is joy. Yet it is. And it is the only real option for emotional well-being. But we must be mature to work this puzzle.

Many clients are not able to take the journey from shame to joy. They are afraid that shame and joy are too distant for them to imagine how they might make such an emotional trip. If this describes our clients, our first task is to spend our energy noticing their strengths, until they are strong enough or our relationship with them is strong enough for us to teach them the skill of processing shame.

On the other hand, our clients might be capable of facing shame head on. It takes courage and emotional strength. If we believe our clients possess this quality, we can help them process shame into joy.

First, we must help our clients through fear of guilt and encourage them to be proud of themselves for being willing to feel guilty. Guilt says nothing about the core of a person, except that the person who feels guilty is capable of love and kindness. This is something we all should want. No one is above making a mistake. An honorable person claims responsibility for her behavior and feels the pain that inspires her to change.

Too often a parent/child interaction might go like this:

Child: I'm sorry I tracked in that mud, Mother.

Parent: Sorry, yes, that's what you are, sorry. Nothing but a sorry, good-for-nothing, except to say, "I'm sorry."

In the above interaction, the mother did not reward the child for claiming responsibility for what he did. Instead, his "I'm sorry" became a tool his mother used to assassinate his character.

The following interaction is preferable:

Child: I'm sorry I tracked in that mud, Mother.

Parent: Thank you for being willing to step up and say, "I'm sorry." That takes courage, and I respect you for that. But your "I'm sorry" doesn't get you off the hook.

Child: I know. I will get the mop and clean up this mess, 'cause I made it.

Parent: Thank you, Son. That's very kind of you. I'm pleased that you responded this way. I'm proud that you are the kind of boy who doesn't offer excuses. He looks at what he has done and takes responsibility. That's character, Son, and it looks like you've got that. I'm proud of you. I am more proud of that than of any "A" you might ever make on a report card!

What we want our children and our clients to learn is what we sometimes see in a basketball game when a player makes a bad pass. As she returns down the court, she says, "My fault." We all admire that person who has broad shoulders strong enough to carry the blame she deserves.

We need strength to feel guilt. If someone pretends to be sorry and doesn't pick up the heavy pain associated with the "I'm sorry," that individual is acting like a manipulative sociopath who has not changed her behavior or point of view when she feels guilty about a particular act. The pain of that guilt eventually will inspire a change in our behavior and attitude. But we must have the courage to feel that pain.

This is what we should help our clients learn: that honor is implicit in guilt. And growth can come from having the courage to feel shame. Feelings of pride and honor are expressions of joy. There is no more satisfying joy than the victory of self-control and personal accountability.

The PRIDE Ritual

I offer my clients the PRIDE ritual as a several-times-daily undertaking. This helps them make healthy shame-processing a habit. This version that follows is different from the one proposed in chapter 9 to combat addiction.

Step 1: <u>P</u>reserve your dignity by moving into the wrong that you did. Do not run away and defend. This makes you look foolish. Embrace the wrong first and confess the sin. There is always something we could have done better that we wish we could do over. Learn from your mistake. Find it, address it, and resolve to tell the person who is hurt why you are sorry.

 Step 2: <u>R</u>eceive and experience the shame. It takes great courage to feel this bad. This feeling, however, is your friend. It will teach you what you need to learn. It will raise your awareness so that you are less likely to make this mistake again. Identify the feeling that you feel now. Feel it for 20 seconds.

Unimportant	Rejected
Devalued	Powerless
Disregarded	Unlovable
Accused	Unfit for Human Contact

 Step 3: <u>I</u>nform yourself of the truth. You made a mistake, but the mistake does not define your soul. At your core, you are a well-intended person who tries to do right. No negative labels define the whole of you. Tell the truth. Answer the question you posed for yourself in the second step (the **R** step). Are you: unimportant, worthy of disregard, unlovable, rightly accused, without value because someone rejects you, powerless, unlovable, or unfit for human contact? The answer is, of course, no. Say no to yourself firmly as the answer to the question. Tell the truth about what you did and who you are. Now, with your shame contained, make amends.

 Step 4: <u>D</u>etect the pride that comes from learning from your mistakes and doing what's right. As you have reminded yourself that you are worthy, valuable, important, powerful, and lovable, and as you have done your best to do the right thing, feel the pride and honor that is a natural consequence of believing in yourself and doing what you believe is right. You have just had the courage to confess whatever you did wrong, feel pain for your wrong, learn and put these feelings in perspective, and, as best you can, do the right thing in the future. You have a right to feel pride in the growth and development that came from the pain of shame.

 Step 5: <u>E</u>ngage life with self-respect.

The PRIDE ritual needs some additional steps when shame has become a prison. When we care too much about what others think and feel ashamed because we cannot please them, pride in the fact that we are caring human beings is not enough to free us from shame. But it is a first step.

Pride in our compassion reminds us that we are the only people capable of balancing our needs with the needs of others. Others can never know us as well as we know ourselves. Our best effort at amends is all that is required. Once offered and rejected it is our task to feel good about our efforts and the internal process that we used to feel compassion and offer a basis for peace. Peace at any price is not peace.

There are two other visible nodes that indicate the resolving relationship between shame and joy. One is in the experience of embarrassment. Embarrassment is a less intense version of shame (Lewis, 1995; Izard, 1972; Tomkins, 1963). Embarrassment is expressed by looking ambivalent and then looking away, accompanied by smiling behavior (Edelman, 1987; Geppert, 1986; Lewis, et al., 1989; Lewis 1995).

Embarrassment is really a question. It asks: "How much shame do I need or do you need me to feel here?". It then proposes an answer by asking another question with a smile: "Can we just laugh about it?" If the answer is "yes" then there is joy and relief. What is said by this emotional expression is, "I made a mistake, but no harm done. Oh, I'm happy that somehow, in my clumsiness, I am able to remain an acceptable companion. That gives me joy."

And there it is again: joy, resolving shame, as embarrassment is resolved successfully.

The second example of this relationship between joy and shame is documented by Nathanson (1992) around the issue of sexual desire. We all feel shame when we have sexual feelings toward another person who we believe will not welcome our interest. To determine whether or not our sexual interest is welcome, we flirt. We look coyly at him or her and remark about something that is attractive about his or her appearance. This is a euphemism for "I want to have sex with you." If our attention seems welcome, we continue to increase the level of our intimate self-disclosures. We might back up when we think we have received a discouraging signal. Courtship rarely proceeds in a straight line. We remain ashamed of our intense sexual desires toward that object, until we discover that our affection and desire is reciprocated. When that happens, it is, "Oh joy, oh joy, Hallelujah!" Again, *joy* is shame's resolution.

Summary and Conclusion

Remember what Craig last said: "How can I look at Enid without guilt, if I can't look at myself in the mirror?" I tried to help Craig answer that question.

"What does Enid see when she looks at herself in the mirror?" I replied. "She sees herself as fat and ugly, a woman who is not able to keep her husband, who is so demanding and greedy that she drove her husband to taking ill-advised risks, and was so bitter when he failed her that she could not forgive him. Her bitterness drove him into another woman's arms. That's what she sees when she looks in the mirror."

"But that's not who she is," Craig said.

"No, it is not. When Enid thinks this way she is indulging in a self-pre-scribed pity party. She did these things, but these things don't accurately define her. Enid's rendition of herself leaves out Enid the comic, Enid the mother, Enid the bold one who went to face Lindsay. We could go on and on."

"Yes, we could," Craig agreed.

"And so we could in saying good things about you," I continued. "It is your job to know who you are, to see yourself clearly, both the good and the bad. Yes, there is bad, but there is more good than bad to Craig. It is your job to know that. It is Enid's job to know that about herself. You made mistakes. Enid did, too, but a mistake is just a mistake. It does not define your soul. I'm a mess. You're a mess, Enid is, too. I have to accept myself and my sins and go on. So do you, so does Enid. That's the job."

"A very tough job for me right now."

"Aren't you proud that you love Enid?"

"Yes, I am," Craig said.

"I assume you love your children," I continued. "Let's imagine that you hurt one of them. How would you wish you felt?"

"I wish I would feel ashamed."

"And that is how you feel about what you did that hurt Enid," I explained. "You feel profoundly ashamed...because you love her. And yet you say you are proud that you love Enid."

"I am."

"Did you expect to go through your married life with Enid and never hurt her, never make a mistake that would cause her pain? Do you have to be so perfect that you can't live with the fact that you made a mistake and you hurt her?"

"I'm beginning to get it, I think," Craig said.

"Do you expect your children to be so perfect in their relationships with you, Enid, their siblings, and their eventual mates? The odds are high that one of them will have an extra-marital affair."

"I hope not," Craig said.

"But if they did, would you despise them for it?"

"No, I would simply expect them to tell the truth and do their best to make amends. That would be enough for me."

"If they did that, would you be proud of them?" I asked.

"Yes, I would indeed. I don't expect them to be perfect. I just expect them to take responsibility for their behavior and fix what can be fixed and make sacrifices to make amends. Whoever can do that is a person of character. I think my children can do that."

"So can Enid."

"Yes, she sure can, and she is doing that. I truly love and respect her for how she has handled this."

"And what about you? Are you proud of yourself for not running off with Lindsay? She would have solved your money worries. You would have had the great sex of a new relationship, maybe a new family, certainly a new life. You turned that down. Are you proud that you hurt when you thought about hurting someone you love, like Enid? Are you proud that you are making amends with Enid and working to rebuild your life together with her?"

"Yes, I am proud of these things."

"When you look in the mirror, I would like you to see a person who screws up from time to time, but when he does, he cares about the hurt he causes. He cares, and he hurts, too, because he has a big heart. He loves so deeply and profoundly that he hurts when he causes pain to those he loves. And because of his big heart and this hurt that he feels, he does whatever he can to learn, change, do better, and sacrifice for healing. That's who I hope you can see."

"I'm beginning to see glimpses of him," Craig said.

"I want you to use this ritual. I think it will help you."

"God knows I need the help."

"It's called the PRIDE technique. You should repeat it one or more times daily."

"Like, take twice a day and call me if you're not feeling better?"

"Sort of," I said.

He did and some weeks later he said, "Boy, I wasn't sure I would ever get out of the hole I dug for myself. That PRIDE technique was a big help. So was church. The PRIDE ritual gave me the same message as one of my minister's sermons. Feeling and confessing shame is a good thing, and the fact that I'm able to do that makes me a person of character. I guess that's true. Enid seems to think so as well, but what's important is that I'm getting it. Practicing that ritual helped."

CHAPTER 11

Surprise/Startle/Wonder
Emotions' Clutch

Surprise/Startle/Wonder Defined

Surprise is another emotion like interest/desire/excitement. The intensity of felt emotion makes a qualitative difference in the emotional expression, from out-of-control startle, to the momentary surprise, to the reflective experience of wonder.

Surprise is one of Ekman's Sacred Seven. It is well researched because of this (Ruffman & Keenan, 1996). We first see it reported in infants of about 6 months old. Surprise throws our body and psyche into neutral (Nathanson, 1990). It clears our minds of other emotions and other thoughts just as a clutch on a standard transmission car takes it out of gear. As the mind's palate is cleansed by surprise, we are asking the questions: what, how, when, or why. Our head tilts to the side. Our eyes squint as if we are trying to see more clearly. We have a blank look on our face, as if the face is alert, asking a question, wondering, not knowing. There has been a violation of what we had expected. A steady state has been interrupted. "What the...?" are the words forming in our mouths.

Surprise can come from a discovery of a wonderful thing that we hadn't expected or from a sudden threat. If we are hoping for something to happen, but afraid that it won't, we are delightfully surprised when it does. Such a surprise will lead us to joy. We can be surprised when things do not go as expected and we are unprepared for what has come to pass. This surprise is likely to lead us to fear or anger.

Surprise needs to be short-lived. Surprise prepares us for a new emotion, just as the clutch prepares the car's engine for a new gear. Left engaged too long, the clutch burns out. Surprise makes way for a fresh start. It announces to us and others that we don't know. We are confused. We are wondering. When in a crisis, we can only afford to be in the state of not-knowing for a short time. We had better get in gear, figure out what it is, and what we feel, if we are to respond effectively.

Startle is the most extreme version of this emotion. It is a sudden jolt of arousal. It fires all our nerves at once. Usually a startle response is not a pleasant experience. But we quickly forget our surprise, and we remember and associate it with the valence, positive or negative, of the emotion that follows.

Wonder is the most steady state of this emotion. It is the basis of awe, mystery, and spiritual experience. It forms the foundation, together with interest, of all curious exploration. Wonder is a chosen surprise.

Surprise is the emotion we feel in response to change. Whether the response is as intense as startle/surprise or merely wonder depends on how much we care about what's going on and how afraid we are at the time. If we are not that aroused and we are not afraid and what's happening doesn't matter to us, a sudden change will make us merely wonder, "What could that be?" (Lang, Bradley, & Cuthbert, 1990).

Clinical Case Study

I first saw Jill when she was 14 years old. Her family was new to Nashville, and she was having a tough time adjusting. She was now 25. She was in a serious relationship, and she came to me for help. This was our conversation:

"His name is Todd," Jill said. "I can't seem to get my arms around him. Oh, that's not what I mean. Trying to work with him is like trying to put your hand on a cloud, while thinking it's a table—for a moment, he's there and then he's not. He doesn't exactly say he's there. He is like an eclipse."

"Well, tell me a story," I said, "so I can have something concrete to work with."

"OK. Well, this reunion, for example," she said. "I told him it's at a Shakespeare festival. He seemed excited . . ."

"No, tell me exactly what you said and he said."

"I said, 'Todd, I'm going to see my friend Jessica at her parents' family reunion. They have it every year at the Utah Shakespeare Festival in Cedar City. Would you like to come?' 'That sounds like fun,' he said. 'I don't know. Maybe I can. Wouldn't it be great? What plays are being performed?'"

"I told him *Merry Wives of Windsor*, *The Merchant of Venice*, Chekov's *Cherry Orchard*, and *Peter Pan*. 'Those are great plays,' he said. 'I would love to go.'"

"He asked me questions about Shakespeare, about Cedar City, about the Troyers, about when was the last time I saw *Peter Pan*. He said he saw himself much like Peter Pan. I assumed he was going. Then, I don't hear from him. Finally, 3 days before I was leaving to go, I called him, and he tells me that he has other plans. He is rafting down a river with some new friends.

"He is the same way about the relationship. He says things like, 'I wonder what it would be like if we were married,' or 'I would love to have kids someday.' 'I wonder what it would be like if we had children together.' Then, other days, he says, 'I'm not sure I can ever handle marriage or kids. I don't know.'"

Jill changed the subject. "Can I talk to you about sex? Can you handle that?"

"I think so," I replied.

"I tell him that for me sex requires a committed relationship. He says he understands. But there's a girl he wants to see in New York, and another one is in Michigan. He then tells me that he loves me and that I turn him on and that he wants to do it. I assume that this means that he understands that doing it would mean that he is committed to keeping sex exclusive to us. He never says that to me. But we do it. He's great, by the way. Then, I don't hear from him for 2 weeks. I find out from a friend that he's gone to New York to visit that girl.

"When he got back, I confronted him. He was clueless. He never promised me anything, he said. Sometimes, he says, he wants to be committed to me and other times he is not sure what he wants. He says he is exploring. He is curious. He wonders about things all the time. He can't stop asking questions about 'what would life be if . . .' He doesn't want to hurt me. He doesn't want to lose me, he says.

"He says that I surprise him when I say I believed he had agreed to something that in his mind he did not. He seems to be constantly surprised or wondering. That's what attracted him to me. He wasn't like other guys who seemed so certain about everything. He believes in magic and miracles. He thinks love is a miracle. And he is waiting for that miracle to pull him into love. He says that maybe I am that miracle. I love it when he talks to me that way.

"Generally, guys know everything, or have a theory or opinion about everything. When Todd hears someone offer an opinion, he just says, 'That's very interesting.' His most direct, in-your-face comment is, 'You think so?' Then, he continues the conversation with another question. When you ask him a direct question, he always says, 'I don't know. What do you think?' He is constantly curious, always asking, always admitting that he doesn't know. Now I've got the confusion disease. I know I want to be with Todd. I just don't know how to make that work."

"Will he come with you to see me?" I wondered.

"I will ask," she replied.

Neurology of Surprise/Startle/Wonder

The startle response is a primitive emotion based in the brainstem. There are two paths for the startle response. One is related to fear. The startle/fear response proceeds through the rostrolateral midbrain. Like anger and fear, the startle/wonder response also proceeds through the caudal neural amygdalofugal pathway. But the rostrolateral midbrain does not mediate startle/wonder (Frankland & Yoemans, 1995).

We associate surprise/startle/wonder primarily with the left hemisphere. The fear/startle response is associated with vocalization, ejaculation, urination, and defecation. The startle/wonder response is associated with assertive behaviors directed toward appetites and desires (Buck, 1999). In the brainstem, the ascending reticular activating system (ARAS) mediates all startle responses (Routtenberg, 1978).

As we move away from startle to surprise and wonder, we know less about how the brain works. Surely the arousal brain systems involved in interest/excitement/desire are also involved in surprise and wonder.

Panksepp (1998) proposes an emotional system that he terms "the expectancy system." In our emotional taxonomy, it would be a combination of interest/excitement/ desire with joy and startle/surprise/wonder. He proposed that dopamine, glutamate, several opiates, several neuropeptides, and neurotensin are involved in that system.

Clearly, a startle/surprise emotion exists. Whether or not wonder is involved is a matter of serious debate and further research. What is clear to me is that some people take on a posture of surprise or not-knowing, hiding behind a constant facade that looks like the blank facial expression of surprise. These people are searchers, inquirers. They don't have to know. But they do have to ask, and they want most subjects to remain open. Knowing would terminate inquiry.

For the purposes of a clinician, what is most important is discovering how and why we cast ourselves in a particular emotional posture and what are the behavioral and psychological correlates of this posture.

The most promising research that links all the states of inquiry from startle to wonder is the work of Lang, Bradley, and Cuthbert (1990). They found that two variables increase the intensity of surprise. The more fearful one is, the more intense the startle response; the more aroused one is, the more intense the startle response. If we are not afraid or not that energized, when a novel stimulus is received, we likely say to ourselves, "I wonder what that is?"

The Physiology of the Startle/Surprise/Wonder Response

The eye blink is to the startle response what the blush is to shame. It is a physiological marker of being startled. Researchers use the eye blink to study the startle response (Lang, Bradley, & Cuthbert, 1990). Studying the startle response, researchers have developed an elaborate amount of information concerning the musculature around the eye. Studies also have linked several other physiological correlates to the startle response and surprise. They are: an increase in heart rate, a short electro-dermal response duration, respiratory irregularity, lowered hand temperature, and higher skin-conductance level (Bradley, Lang, & Cuthbert, 1993).

The Intelligence of the Startle/Surprise/Wonder Response

Clearly, we cannot attach much intelligence to this emotion. The only positive thing about this confused state is that in this state we know that we don't know and we ask questions.

The Negative Consequences of Startle/Surprise/Wonder

Certainly, negative consequences occur when we do not have a startle response. People who suffer from epilepsy and depression have a diminished startle response. The distinguishing feature of catatonic schizophrenia is flat affect and a severely diminished startle response (Dawson, Hazlett, Filion, & Nuechterlein, 1993). Nathanson (1992) claims that there is little or no downside to having an excessive amount of surprise.

I contend that startle/surprise/wonder has a dark side. People can use surprise and confusion to be manipulative. We all have seen a person hang on to that startled look long after it was genuine response. That person may be feigning surprise and confusion to avoid responsibility or to get others to have sympathy or feel guilty. It is one of the many ways for a person to act passive-aggressively.

Passive-aggressive behavior describes behavior in which by doing nothing, appearing to be surprised, confused, and unaware, we can avoid taking responsibility for our behavior and induce others to do our work for us. As we appear surprised and confused, scratching our head and saying, "I don't know what happened," we cannot participate; we withhold our energy and resources. This behavior punishes others, for instance, those who need us to pitch in with the community project, and helps us avoid blame.

As a child, didn't we all play this game with our parents at one time or another? We wanted something that we couldn't have. We put on that vacant surprised and possibly hurt look and asked, "Why, Mommy?" or "Why not, Daddy?" Our parents would explain, and we would respond with the same look and same question, "Why?" This game could go on for hours. We were looking for an explanation that we could rebut. We kept the pressure on our parents, until they tripped up and gave us something that we could argue with, so that we could change their minds. This child's game usually lasts as long as a parent's patience.

Often the posture of confusion and surprise is a response of the powerless to the powerful. For example, the servant says to the master, "You, Master, are so wise and competent. You know all, and I know nothing. What could this be? I don't know how to do this?" The master is powerless in the face of this line of conversation.

Imagine a second scene. The master looks down in a ditch in which his servant stands holding a shovel. "Master," says the servant, "I don't know how to use a shovel." The scene then changes because of the servant's not-knowing.

Move to the next scene. The master is in the ditch, digging with the shovel, and the servant (out of the ditch and scratching his head) looks down at his master and says, "You sure dig a good ditch, Master. I don't know how to do that."

Not-knowing sets up those who want to be the expert. Many of us do not tolerate surprise and confusion well. We always pretend to know and never appear confused. We volunteer or compete for authority roles. We answer-givers want to assume the authority position. Those who enjoy not-knowing manage us with ease.

In the Southern United States, where I grew up, and in Shakespeare's Elizabethan England, women and servants shrewdly played the surprised role. One can hear Scarlett O'Hara saying, "Well, I do declare. I didn't know that. How smart you are, Rhett Butler!"

The problem with being dependent on the not-knowing posture is how it affects our self-esteem. Yes, it gains power by giving power away. It is seductive and attractive. But sometimes we can begin to believe that we don't know. We can begin to depend on the charity of others and avoid knowing what we do know, thus avoiding self-determination. We are constantly in the control of someone else, sucking up to the most powerful people we can so that they can protect us.

The consequences of this posture are well stated by the many biographers of Marilyn Monroe. She was afraid to know what she knew or how she felt. She hid behind a seductive question mark to keep from having to know or be known. The result was low self-esteem, self-hatred, and suicide.

The Positive Consequence of Startle/Surprise/Wonder

Being curious and inquisitive is obviously a good thing. We all know what can happen when we concoct a theory before all questions have been asked and answered. Startle/surprise/wonder is an essential ingredient to the inquiry. It is part of the foundation of problem-solving, spiritual development, play, and creativity.

Children love to have conditions change so that for a second or two they don't know what's going on; they wonder if they should be afraid or sad or angry, only to discover that no there is no threat. The joy of laughter follows surprise when they discover they are safe. That's the basis of peek-a-boo and hide-and-seek. Surprise is an essential element of play and entertainment. It's even a basic dramatic device used by authors, playwrights, and screenwriters to surprise readers, audiences, and filmgoers, perhaps scare them a little only to relieve them later of their fears.

As adults, do we believe in magic or miracles? Do we wonder if there are spiritual dimensions that we humans cannot comprehend? Do we have faith that a spiritual dimension exists? If we answer "yes" to any of these questions, we are honoring the emotion of surprise. We are inviting the universe to surprise us with events beyond our comprehension. Because we have a faith of some sort, we can explain these surprises as miracles or magic.

All major religions have prayers that implicitly or explicitly include a statement similar to the following:

> Dear (Allah, God, Shiva, and so forth),
> We don't understand your ways. We can't comprehend your power. We can't even begin to grasp you or your will. Help us search for your truth with open minds. Give us the courage to wait to be surprised and startled by your direction and the miracles that we know will come from you.
>
> Amen

Surprise is essential to the celebration of mystery and faith.

The Not-Knowing Pose

This is the classical psychoanalytic therapist posture. The analyst refuses the expert role and holds on to not-knowing and wondering. The purpose of this is to keep the analysand (otherwise known as the client) a bit frustrated and continuing her exploration into knowing herself.

Visual artists often talk about how startled they are to find something in their work that they didn't intend. At first, they might direct their anger inward. They consider what they did as a mistake, and they have the impulse to destroy their work and start again. Then, they step back and look at what they did. They are often surprised to see a brilliant new direction in what they once had considered a mistake. Suddenly, their mistake is transformed into something wonderful—something beyond what they could have imagined. Their art seems to talk back to them, surprising them with new ideas, directions, and forms.

Many artists are not only open to these surprises; they also talk about these moments as opportunities for dialogue between them and their medium. These surprises can be the most interesting and enjoyable aspects of an artist's work.

Writers often talk about writing and becoming surprised by what their characters say. They tell of books they have outlined to follow a certain direction. Yet, in the middle of writing the book, they are stunned when one of their characters says words that the writer did not intend to write. They write what they hear their characters say. They keep writing, not knowing what will come next, surprised by each new paragraph as the book takes on a new, unplanned direction.

We would not have many of our modern scientific discoveries without surprise. Consider bacteriologist Andrew Fleming. He was throwing away culture plates that had been contaminated with mold, when he was surprised to see something he had never noticed: a halo or ring of clear, bacteria-free medium around each island of mold. His surprise led to the development of the first antibiotic: penicillin (Nathanson, 1992).

Surely we want to play, wonder about life's mysteries, and be open to seeing reality in an entirely new way. Surprise is an emotion we want to have and enjoy often. But we want surprise to last for a short period, and followed by awareness and a new emotion appropriate to the new circumstance.

Children and Surprise

Children naturally enjoy surprise. As infants, everything is new. Surprise is followed by discovery and awareness. Because children have a short attention span, they welcome surprise as a diversion. Children in the company of their parents usually enjoy a surprise, unless they are frightened by it.

We can use surprise to offer a child the opportunity to change her mood. Surprise/startle can wipe the mind clean of *what was* and open it to *what can be*. If we offer a child a surprise when she is sad, if she is ready to let go of her sadness, she might exchange sadness for another emotion following her surprise. On the other hand, the child might reject our attempt to surprise her and persist in holding on to her old mood.

Some children are born with an acutely sensitive startle response. They jump at any sudden changes in their environment. When a child is easily startled, we must instill in her faith that good can follow a surprise. She needs play activity that includes surprise followed by pleasure, security, and mastery.

If a child associates surprise only with danger and fear, surprise will be a source of fear and pain for the rest of that child's life (Panksepp, 1993). That would be especially harmful to her, because her acutely sensitive startle response is not likely to change as she grows older. Surprise is likely to be a daily emotional event. If surprise always means danger and hurt, surprise will create fear. When we predict that fear and danger will follow surprise, frequently that prophecy becomes self-fulfilling. When surprise merges with fear, the result often is paranoia.

Life is full of change and surprises. We can never anticipate everything. The difference between one who thrives in life and one who does not is how that individual responds to the surprises that are part of change. If we are able to see opportunity in change, we are likely to make lemonade from lemons, silver from the linings of clouds. Our goal should be to help our clients and children associate surprise with excitement and anticipation. Change then will become a good thing. We all want to have this faith in life, in surprises, and in ourselves.

Adults and Surprise

As adults, we assume that experience has taught us to predict and anticipate changes in our circumstances. Predicted and anticipated changes are not surprises for us. We prepare for winter. We slow down at yellow traffic lights. We save for our retirement.

Often, we enjoy the role of expert—one who can predict what will happen next in our field of expertise. A lawyer can predict how courts will decide by studying precedents in case law. An orthopedic surgeon can predict how a bone will heal and how long it will take by examining x-rays. A hydroelectric engineer can predict how much concrete will be needed for a dam to raise the level of a river into a lake by relying on calculations.

To experts, surprises are the enemy. Mastery means control. As adults, we can become addicted to mastery and control and strive to be master of everything. Of course, that's not possible. Surprise will find us, no matter how expert we are or how prepared we might be.

Adults can have pathological responses to surprise. We can become so addicted to control that we hate surprises. A surprise birthday party can be a trauma. A surprise promotion can be unwelcome. A new car bought by a spouse for her mate can be unappreciated because the recipient was not prepared.

For those who are addicted to control, children present an almost insurmountable challenge. Children are unpredictable. Controlling them too tightly only increases explosions and conflict. Perhaps children are God's antidote for adults who need to control. If that's their job, they do it well by giving their parents a constant supply of surprises. We can only hope that we, as their parents, can help resolve their surprises into delight. We can only hope that we, as therapists, can help our clients see opportunities in crises.

When we associate surprise with fear and failure, we become chronic cynics. We become risk-averse. We tend to avoid people and see change as danger.

In our minds, change and challenge may only present a threat. Because life is full of surprise and change, we live in fear of the future. Whatever sense of humor we have is dark and sarcastic.

A pessimist is an individual who hides his talents under a bushel and puts his money in a mattress. His pessimism might have roots in his childhood, when as a child, surprises brought disappointment.

Surprise and change will always be a part of our clients' lives just as it is part of our own. We can't protect our clients from these surprises, but we can help them prepare by reminding them that surprise and change always bring another chance. We can encourage them to associate laughter with surprise, thus giving clients a sense of humor that they can use to transform surprise into fun. Just as fear begets fear, faith begets faith. Just as the self-fulfilling prophecy of danger creates danger, so does the self-fulfilling prophecy of success create success.

Of course, we all want to be capable of being surprised. Our task as therapists is to help our clients see their own strengths so that they can develop faith and cope with the changes that are implicit in a surprise.

Post-traumatic Stress Disorder and Surprise/Startle

Post-traumatic stress is an extreme version of pessimism. Individuals suffering from this condition cannot trust people, jobs, or themselves. Because surprise to them means injury or death, they find it difficult to understand what really is happening when they are surprised in an environment that is relatively benign (Orr, Lasko, Arieh, & Pitman, 1995). They have difficulty believing that change and surprises are not catastrophes.

As an example, surprises in war are mostly painful. One after another, they negatively bombard soldiers. And yet the job of a soldier is to push forward into the source of these surprises that come in the form of bombs and bullets exploding about them, friends losing limbs and dying, and the reality that a mortal wound might be their next surprise. Naturally, for these individuals post-traumatic stress is a common consequence.

An abusive marriage can create the same fear and distrust. And, when children experience a painfully traumatic surprise—divorce or the sudden death of a parent—they feel as if the bottom has dropped out of their world, and they retreat into fear.

When we are constantly surprised and all of those surprises contain fear, danger, and stress, we begin to see life as filled with danger. We have difficulty believing that safety exists. This is post-traumatic stress disorder. It is a disease of surprise/startle. Therapists must be committed to work for a long time to help these clients again develop faith in their futures.

Finding Strength in Our Response to Surprise

Most of us have a characteristic response to surprise. Many of us have a strong need to know. We don't tolerate the question, "What's going on here," for very long. Ambiguity and uncertainty are threatening. For us, the questions posed by surprise are answered quickly. I call those who respond this way to surprise "theory builders."

Others of us enjoy the mystery that surprise creates. Rather than finding the answers to the questions posed by surprise, we hang on to their ambiguity as a protective cover. The term I use for those who enjoy the question is "seekers."

As we observe our clients' responses to surprise, we probably can determine whether they are quick to find the answer or whether they enjoy the mystery of the question. There is nothing wrong with either personality style.

We must help our clients see their strengths. If they are theory builders, their strengths include creativity, imagination, a sense of mastery, and confidence. If our clients are seekers, our job is to help them see the strengths of that personality style—of curiosity, imagination, interest in others, tolerance, and appreciation for the quest. Theory builders can come out of the clouds and act on the best available theory so that they can move forward, while seekers need help to commit to one plan of action and see it through. Seekers can keep the inquiry open, making room for everyone to speak and for as many potential answers as possible, while theory builders close off debate and often move prematurely into action.

Therapists should encourage the theory builders to admit when they are wrong and to return to surprise and the quest for a new theory. And therapists should praise seekers for the courage to make a commitment and stay the course.

Once our clients discover their personality style, praise the strengths they display in managing and using surprise. And when they act against their personality type, praise them for trying a new approach to surprise.

Transforming Startle to Wonder

Passive clients easily can become the pawn of change. Surprise can make them a victim or they can use surprise to be a co-creator of change. Whether our clients become a victim or co-creator depends on their attitudes toward surprise. Since change and surprise are a part of life, we need to help clients learn how to use surprise as an opportunity for creativity. If they are afraid of surprise, they will freeze when they are startled and remain paralyzed until the familiar returns. If they are excited by surprise and curious about what surprise is bringing them, they will become a co-creator. Obviously, we want to help clients take advantage of change and look for the opportunities that come with surprise.

Consider my client, John, an accountant for the local utility company. He saw the trend for local utilities to downsize and merge. He is afraid that one day he will be surprised by a pink slip. He is afraid to go to work for fear that this will be the day.

John: In my current job, I've got benefits. I make good money. I can feel the downsizing coming and the ax falling on my neck.

Therapist: Have you asked your boss about it?

John: No, I'm afraid he will use my question as an opportunity to let me go.

Therapist: This is really frightening. Each day you face this fear? What a burden!

John: Yes it is, and I'm exhausted by it.

Therapist: Do you like your job?

John: No, but it's all I've ever known. I've worked there for 20 years.

Therapist: What would you like to do if you were free to do whatever?

John: I don't know.

Therapist: Well, let's wonder together. I would like to play golf. I've dreamed of being a professional golfer. What about you?

John: I used to imagine being a fireman or a baseball player. Recently I've gotten into computer games. It might be fun to design those. I've dreamed of being the CEO of our company. Fat chance.

Therapist: Let's take the CEO dream. Imagine you had to design the plan for downsizing.

John: I've thought of that. Computers could eliminate several accounting jobs, as well as many jobs in reception and personnel. I know what jobs I would consolidate if I were CEO.

Therapist: Since you know it's coming, why don't you begin to plan for it? Put together a resume. Take courses in programming computer games. Precipitate the crisis. That's what they call it in business school. Go to your boss and tell him you have some ideas about downsizing and job consolidation. Join him in solving his problem. You know he hates to think about these decisions alone. Become the architect of change instead of its victim. Imagine. Play with the possibilities. Plan for a new job. Then, who knows, you may be the person kept and not the one let go. By that time you may be ready to leave with opportunities elsewhere.

John: I've never thought of this situation as an opportunity. I hate my job really. It would take some nerve, but it's better than being afraid every time I get in the car to go to work. Anything is better than the dread I've been feeling. Surprise my boss before he surprises me. I like that idea.

It can be fun to encourage our clients to use change instead of being its victim. Imagining ways to use change can be a game. No answer is wrong. All answers have elements of the right answer. Clients' imaginations are engaged. This search for a plan of action becomes exciting. Surprise becomes an opportunity for play. As we follow along with our clients, we therapists don't have to go directly to the right answer. We can travel together with them around the answer. We can pretend with lots of possibilities. The search for the answer becomes a journey to the zoo or even to France. The obvious first answer might not be the answer when we finish.

Surprise gives us and our clients an opportunity for an exciting, safe, and interesting adventure of imagination.

In our example, surprise becomes a challenging opportunity to wonder and create, rather than merely a danger to fear. I write this as my wife and I travel to a church retreat. She predicts the retreat will be filled with surprises. She wonders what they will be. As she talks, she says we might meet new people; we might have fun; we might be inspired. This could happen or that could happen; things we never imagined will happen.

Her attitude contrasts with mine. I know what will happen. I will be anxious and feel clumsy and awkward. I will compete for the group's attention with other men. I will become a bore. I won't make new friends. People will find me a harrumphing curmudgeon. I hope by the time we get to the retreat that my wife can fill me full of wonder, curiosity, and imaginative, playful creativity. Good luck, Marietta.

Resolving Surprise/Startle/Wonder

The function of this emotion is to be easily resolved into any other emotion. All emotions are appropriate next steps from surprise. *Anger* can follow surprise when there is a threat. *Sadness* can follow surprise when the surprise is interpreted as a loss. *Joy* can follow surprise when surprise comes to mean success or achievement. *Fear* like anger can follow surprise. But we can get stuck in fear being associated with surprise, and that can keep us from finding opportunities to be creative with the surprise of change.

For our clients who are captured by the pose of not-knowing, I have developed another four-step ritual that they might practice daily. The object of the ritual is to use a stimulus to inquire and the process of inquiry to get to an answer and then to make a commitment to knowing and using the answer produced by our inquiry. This process takes us from wondering and not-knowing to the joy of mastery, knowing, and faith.

I use the acronym **SEEK**.

 Step 1: Surprise occurs, and we ask the what, why, how, or when questions that begin our inquiry.

 Step 2: Engage our imaginations to play with all the possible answers, searching and being curious and interested. Do not solve the puzzle of your surprise. Keep asking. Keep wondering. Develop as many answers as possible. I want others to wonder with you. But do not take too much time. Don't hide in the questions.

 Step 3: Evaluate the answers that come from our imaginative play. This is a process of filtering out the answers that do not seem to fit. We use our judgment in choosing an answer, closing down our inquiry and selecting what we believe to be our best choice.

 Step 4: Keep your promise. Commit and act on the answer. Here, we believe in the process we went through to get our answer. This is the place to act as if we know. We stay the course. Move forward with the certainty of the master we have become in this process until we are surprised again. The surprise must be a significant one. Don't let a small detail derail your plan. If the surprise is a significant one, repeat the SEEK process.

Summary and Conclusion

Todd returned with Jill the next week.

"How can I help?" I began.

"I can't get Todd to tell me whether or not we have a future," Jill began.

"I'm the curious sort," Todd said. "I don't see why we have to trap ourselves into a future we know nothing about. I don't see why Jill can't just enjoy the moment and let the future take care of itself."

"So, if I want to find out how you feel about me, I have to withdraw or make you jealous," Jill said. "I hate that. I refuse to play games. This is who I am, Todd. You see what you get. I want to be with you. Why can't you respond and tell me whether or not you want me?"

"Courtship, like it or not, is a game," I said. "Both people play the game, coming together, then going apart, coming together, then going apart. You learn a lot about each other in the courtship dance. When we prematurely end courtship, serious problems come to the relationship later when the stakes are much higher. I remember once saying to a girl exactly what you said. I told her my life story, including all its tragedies. I exposed to her what I thought my strengths and weaknesses were. And then I proclaimed my love for her. She listened quietly to my soliloquy, and then responded. 'David,' she said, 'I don't really know you.' 'Yes, you do,' I protested. 'Well, perhaps,' she said. 'Maybe I know more about you than I'm ready to know. What I'm sure about is how I feel. I feel very uncomfortable. It is like I have been bought and paid for by what you consider the courage you have to share so much. To me, it feels like blackmail. Now I am supposed to reciprocate, and I'm not ready. I don't want to tell you my life story. How can you love me? You don't know me. We haven't played tennis together. I don't know how you can handle losing a point to me. You don't know how I behave when I'm mad. I'm not ready for a serious relationship with you, and your wanting it won't make me ready.'"

"That's how I feel," Todd said. "I love being with Jill, but she wants a commitment and I'm not ready for that. I think Jill hates the awkwardness of getting to know one another and the stupid things that we do. I think she wants to get that part over, papering over it with sex, solidifying this infant stage before it finds its legs. I'm not sure she loves me so much as she wants to get to the next stage of her life, and I am the guy she's with when she's ready. I know I am not ready. I'm not sure I ever will be."

"Then why did you come today?" I wondered.

"Because I'm curious. I've never been to a therapist before. I like to try new things. I get bored easily, and I'm always up for something different. I love new places, new things, new ideas, and new people. I like change. That is one of the reasons I'm not sure I'm marriage material."

"Jill," I said. "In a relationship there is always a certain amount of doubt and fear versus a certain amount of faith and commitment. Imagine these were two substances in two bowls, one bowl filled with faith and commitment and the other with fear and doubt. If you reach into the faith and commitment bowl and you possess all of that substance, what is left for Todd?"

"I see," Jill said. "He will have only fear and doubt, and that's what he will express while I am trying to convince him to let go of his fear and doubt and come with me into commitment."

"Yes, that's right. But since you have taken all the commitment—and all relationships have commitment and doubt—then Todd will hold on to the doubt. He can only get commitment if you give up some of it and reach into the fear/doubt bowl."

"Hence the game," Jill said.

"Yes," Todd agreed. "I kind of like the game. I enjoy the unknown. I like surprises. You said you like that about me."

"Yes," Jill said. "I do. I find your curiosity very charming. But I wonder if you can ever dip into the commitment bowl?"

"Perhaps you are right," Todd replied. "I don't know."

"Your curiosity is becoming less attractive to me now. Being mysterious as you are, full of curiosity and wonder about life, is attractive. But it is not real, is it? There is nothing for me to join. There is no ground under your feet. When I ask you a question, Todd, you seem pleased to answer, 'I don't know.' I wonder if you will ever be willing to claim what you know."

"Those are harsh words," Todd said. "People have seemed to like my curiosity and wonder. If you don't, I think someone else will."

"Yes," I said, "But, Todd, who would want to partner with Peter Pan?"

"Wendy," Todd said.

"But only for so long," Jill said.

Todd and Jill left both a bit shaken. Todd called me the next day and wanted to see me by himself.

"What can I do about this Peter Pan thing? My mother says the same thing to me. 'You're charming, Todd,' she says, 'but what is there to you after that? You are a jack-of-all-trades with your questions. But before you really work to learn something substantial and useful you get bored. So you are the master of none.' Is there something I can do about this?"

"Well," I replied, "As a matter of fact, you can try this ritual I have designed for people who has trouble knowing and claiming what they know. You practice it daily, or more. It will only take 5 minutes."

Todd said, "I'll give it a try."

He came back 6 weeks later and said, "I tried that SEEK ritual. I used it a couple of times a day. You were right. It was designed for me. As I used it, I began to know things. Among the things I began to know were things about myself. I admitted to myself that I loved to paint and sculpt more than anything else. I was afraid to know that, because I knew my parents would not approve. My not knowing kept the doors open but did not expose me to my parents' disapproval.

"I also learned that I do not want to be with Jill. What I want to commit to is my art. I'm going to use the $25,000 inheritance from my grandfather and go to Paris to pursue my career as an artist, well, not really an artist, probably a food server who paints. I do want to have a committed relationship, but that would be with a woman who understands and supports my commitment to art.

"I appreciate your help. I'm not sure my parents do. They were paying your bill, and from now on, I'm sure I can't afford you."

"I would love to see you when you come back from Paris. Call me and make an appointment. I will charge something you can afford."

CHAPTER 12

Fatigue/Relaxation/Sleep/Trance
Emotions' Anesthesia

Fatigue/Relaxation/Sleep/Trance Defined

Fatigue/Relaxation/Sleep/Trance (FRST) is probably the most controversial emotion to be nominated to our list of basic emotions. I defended its choice in chapter 1.

This emotion provides rest and renewal after the others have depleted us of our energy and attention. Using FRST, we can:

- be desperate to close our eyes and sleep and yet remain awake;
- stab our arm with nails and report feeling no pain;
- be in an insoluble crisis one day and, after a good night's sleep, solve the problem the next day;
- be awake, our eyes open, staring into space and be somewhere else in our minds.

I am sure that there will be many critics of my choice of FRST as a basic emotion. I can hear them saying that these states—fatigue, rest, sleep, and trance—are each very distinct states, each with its own set of brain patterns and neurohormones.

While there may be different brain waves with each state, the same parts of the brain are more or less involved. The same is true of the neurohormones; more or less, they are the same. That is what is confusing about this emotion, the more or less. FRST is the obverse of interest/desire/excitement. Just as there are different levels of arousal, there are different levels of rest. FRST—interest/desire/excitement and surprise/startle/wonder—have this quality of being a dimension, not just on or off. These three emotions often provide the subtext for other emotions. They can serve to amplify fear, anger, joy, shame, and disgust or to moderate and lessen the intensity of these emotions.

Fatigue, relaxation, sleep, and trance are different aspects of rest. They overlap one another, and they serve to create a frame for each other. "I was relaxing. I was not asleep." Or, "I am tired, but I'm paying attention." "My eyes are closed, but I'm not asleep. I heard what you said." Or, "I'm sorry I know I was looking right at you, but I wasn't paying attention." These statements suggest the various levels of rest, each different from the other.

Fatigue is a drive like hunger. Fatigue's focus is sleep, or, at the very least, rest. When we are fatigued, our bodies ache for sleep. We are already half asleep. When we give ourselves permission to close our eyes, sleep quickly will come over us. Relaxation is when our eyes are closed. Our brain waves are alpha waves. We are not asleep. We are not awake. We are almost dreaming, but not quite. In sleep, our eyes close. We lose consciousness. Our brains follow predictable patterns, moving from one stage of sleep to the other, then the other, and so forth, until the sleep cycle is complete.

Most of us go through the cycle twice in a night (Cantero, Atienza, Gomez, & Salas, 1999). In the first stage of sleep, we dream. While we sleep, the parasympathetic nervous system is engaged.

During sleep, our muscles are generally relaxed, except during dream sleep or alpha-wave sleep when sometimes our muscles can contract or our hearts race in response to dream images. Our organs are renewed (Strecker, et al., 1999). Sleep is clearly a different state from awake.

That is not true for the trance. The trance is like relaxation, except that during the trance, our eyes are open. Our brain waves tend toward alpha waves (Cantero, et al.,1999). We are in a daydream. Our brains are entranced by a storyteller, movie, play, tennis match, music, or an imaginary fantasy.

The state of trance involves renewal of the body. It informs us that we need rest, relaxation, or sleep. Or, it transports us into our daydreams and imaginations, where our minds need to be turned off and all matters of consequence set aside. Our eyes long to close and surrender to sleep.

Rest renews our bodies and our minds. It has its own facial expressions, its own biochemical brain chemistry, and its own neurological brain-wave patterns. It is an important physical state that our bodies must express.

Fatigue is our body's signal that we need rest now. Without rest, we will lose our sanity and our physical health. Each day, therefore, our body needs to spend a significant time at rest. Relaxation is effective rest, but not deep sleep. The trance also is restful, but our eyes remain open. In sleep, we dream and lose consciousness. Our bodies are renewed and nurtured during sleep.

Clinical Case Study

If this medicine is good for my clients, certainly it is for me as well. I should take some of my own medicine. This is an occasion when I did.

It is August as I write this. My wife, Marietta, and I are on vacation. We had the conversation while we were strolling on Main Street in Park City, Utah.

"David," Marietta said, "I don't want to go on another vacation with you when you are writing a book."

"But Marietta," I protested, "I love to write, and vacation is the only time I have to do it."

"I know, and that is why I have tolerated it this long."

"So, what's the deal with being on vacation with me while I'm writing?"

"It's not so much the writing," Marietta replied. "I can entertain myself while you write for 2 or 3 hours. It is when we are together. Like right now, what were you thinking about?"

"I was thinking about the story and the characters I would write about to introduce my next chapter."

"I knew that. You know how I knew that? It's because you are in a trance. Your mind is not here with me. It's off with your characters. You aren't having a conversation with me. You are talking with them in your trance, and when I speak to you, it's like I'm interrupting something really important. You seem startled by my comments, put off that you have to pay attention to me."

"It's not that bad."

"Oh, you don't know," Marietta protested. "As long as you are writing something, that is where your mind is, off in your imagination, in your trance somewhere, having fun with someone, not me."

"I love my imagination. I don't get much of a chance to use it. As a boy, I used to sit by the floor furnace doing nothing. Family members would pass me in the hall. 'Are you all right, David?' they would ask. Of course, I was. I was warm by the floor furnace, and I was lost in a trance, being a cowboy, Roy Rogers or Lash LaRue. Lash LaRue was my favorite. Why is that so bad?"

"It's not bad for you, David. It's just bad for anyone who wants to be with you and have you be with them. For me it's like being the sober one when everybody around me is drunk or stoned. It's like you have left me."

"I haven't left you."

"Yes, you have, or you might as well have. Were you abused as a child? You seem to run away from me into your imagination when you have no stress. Am I that difficult? Am I so awful that you have to run away from me?"

"No, of course not. What are you saying?"

To be continued.

The Neurology of FRST

If the brain has an "on" switch that arouses the body and if the wiring for that on switch is a part of two emotions—interest and surprise—what do we say about the switch that turns the body off? And when the body is off, what do we call that state?

Buck (1999) and Lindsley (1951, 1957) both propose that the brain has an arousal system. It consists of the ascending reticular activating system (ARAS). This circuitry comprises fibers and cell bodies in the core of the brainstem, extending from the spinal cord to the thalamus (Bremer, 1935). The system acts as a stimuli filter (Lindsley, 1957). It will not turn on the body if a stimulus is weak or repetitive.

Does it not follow that perhaps weak and repetitive stimuli—a mother's heartbeat, lullaby, chant, mantra, familiar song—can be a signal to turn the system off? Sounds like these can turn on a relaxation response that might become sleep.

A segment of the ARAS crucial to sleep regulation is the pontive tegmentum (PT) and, even more specific, the nucleus pontus oralis (NPO) located in the pontive tegmentum. The NPO is especially rich in cholinergic, glutamatergic, catachlomnergic, histaminergic, and GABA receptors. The dorsal raphe nucleus (DRN), the adjacent lateral dorsal (LDT), and the peduncleoponteris tegmental nucleus (PPT) are especially relevant to the production of the first level of sleep termed rapid-eye-movement (REM) sleep or alpha brain-wave sleep (Xi, Morales, & Chase, 1999).

Recent research on spiritual consciousness and the brain confirms much of this speculation. Single photon emission computer tomography machines (SPECT) have been used to photograph the brains of Catholic nuns in meditative prayer and Tibetan Buddhist monks during their meditative practice (D'Aquili & Newberg, 1999). The SPECT revealed that the orientation area of the brain, or the parietal lobe, disengaged during meditation along with the part of the brain that has the awareness of self and a sense of time or the temporal lobe. The SPECT revealed that the frontal lobe which is linked to attention and concentration is engaged.

Researchers (Austin 1998; Newberg & D'Aquili, 1999; Persinger, 2002) contend that the hippocampus acts like a neurological traffic signal to amygdala, the parietal lobe and the temporal lobe, while sending the flow of neurons on the frontal lobe.

These researchers and others have made these discoveries as they searched for the neurology of spiritual experiences. One example concerns what people call an out-of-body experience. In a general trance, the whole temporal lobe is turned off. Persinger (2002) believes that in an out-of-body experience the left temporal lobe is turned on, while the right temporal lobe is turned off.

In the trance that comes from ritualistic drumming, dancing, or chanting, the brain's arousal system is intensely activated while the parietal lobes (the orientation centers) are deactivated, as in deep quiet meditation. In the trance, since our bodies have lost the ability to know where the self begins and where it leaves off, we experience a sense of oneness with all that is.

This implies that there may be many variations on the trance. There is much to be learned, but current research on the spiritual experience of the brain reinforces the idea of the trance as a basic human emotion (Graffin, Ray, & Lundy, 1995).

The same neurohormones that depress the body and inhibit arousal contribute to sleep. They are low levels of norepinephrine (NA), serotonin (5-H7), oxytocin (OXY) and dopamine (DA); high levels of corticotrophin-releasing factor (CRF), peptide neuro-transmitters; monoamine oxidase (MAO); and substance P, the carrier of the pain message (Panksepp, 1986).

The most important neurohormone to the regulation of sleep are GABA hormones. These neurohormones—$GABA_A$ and $GABA_B$—are inhibitory factors in the brain involved in shutting down arousal (Chase, Morales, & Xi, 1999). Also serotonin and the growth hormone-releasing hormone (GHRH) appear to reduce the brain's level of serotonin with each descending level of the sleep cycle (Strecker, et al., 1999). As serotonin decreases, acetylcholine (ACH) increases, especially promoting REM sleep or alpha sleep.

As we age, sleep becomes more difficult. Antonijevic (Antonijevic, et al., 2000) suggested that this occurs because of a decrease in GHRH in our body, as we age. They found that in men that this hormone especially enhanced stage-two sleep, or slow-wave sleep. In women, this hormone had the opposite effect.

Studies of the various levels of sleep are widely known. Three levels of consciousness have been meticulously documented through electroencephalographic (EEG) techniques. The first level of consciousness is wakefulness (W); the second, rapid-eye-movement sleep (REM sleep) or alpha-wave sleep; the third, slow-wave sleep (SWS), or beta-wave sleep (Miller, et al., 1999).

Most research has focused on REM sleep, because it is such a coherent and distinctive sleep pattern. REM sleep alternates with slow-wave sleep, creating a sleep cycle. Apparently, this cycle repeats itself two or three times during a night's rest (Cantero, Atienza, & Salas, 1999).

Slow-wave sleep has had less research attention. Steriade and Amzica (1998) documented three different rhythms of sleep during slow-wave sleep: spindle, 7-14 Hz; delta, 1-4 Hz; and slow oscillation <1 Hz. They found evidence that there was an orderly appearance of these rhythms during slow-wave sleep. It appeared to be associated with a progressive increase in cortcothalmic coherence of sleep rhythms. They speculated that during slow-wave sleep, our brains reorganize and specify circuits to consolidate memory traces that were recorded stimuli during wakefulness.

The Physiology of FRST

During FRST, the body rests. The parasympathetic system in the autonomic nervous system becomes engaged. This turns on the nurturing and renewal systems of the body's internal organs. The heart rate slows during sleep, blood pressure decreases, breathing slows, and healing and renewal occurs. During sleep, the eyes are closed. During REM sleep, the eyes move back and forth. When the body is relaxed, alpha brain waves can occur while the body is awake and the eyes open.

The Intelligence of FRST

Clearly, our mind is not at our disposal during this emotion. Perhaps it is being enriched and renewed by rest, just as is the body. Of course, the species cycle of exercise followed by rest has a genetic intelligence but not a person-specific intelligence. There are many reports of people going to sleep with a question or problem and waking with the answer. But we cannot expect or command our minds to do this work during sleep. Perhaps sleep can provide wisdom, but not conscious intelligence.

The Negative Consequences of FRST

We use FRST on many occasions to avoid reality or to avoid painful feelings. When we use FRST as a defense, it can become a trap that keeps us from growing and learning.

We often use FRST as a way to avoid things we do not want to face. Thus FRST can become a component of sadness and depression. For example, we can become so sad that we want to go to sleep so that we won't feel so sad. Or, we can become so afraid of work (or school or whatever) that we cling to sleep, past the time to go to work. When we awake, we are relieved that it is too late and glad our avoidance technique worked. Some who use sleep this way can sleep 18 hours a day.

Staying asleep for long periods of time can feed on itself. Lack of exercise or activity forces us to lose muscle tone and stamina, and we become so out of shape that we easily tire. Too much sleep helps us to avoid life's challenges, which makes us even more afraid, thus creating a cycle of procrastination, depression, and fatigue.

Rarely do children experience pathological fatigue in this way, but it is common among college students and older adults.

Many people use the trance in a similar way. This can manifest in attention deficit disorder (ADD), when our minds wander from what we wish to be paying attention to. It is what we mean when we say we are bored. The mind tends to shut down and go into a trance if the stimuli we are receiving are weak (not relevant to us) or repetitive ("I've got it already—shut up."). When we can't speak up, when we are bored and forced to listen to a speaker and endure his irrelevant, repetitive, and monotonous talk, what else is there to do but allow our minds to wander?

This, of course, is not healthy for us. It is not good for speakers to lose their audiences, and it results in poor communication and damages relationships.

If we use a trance or develop a delusional system in a dialogue with our imaginations, we might disconnect from reality and become lost in our own world. This can become part of intense paranoia or schizophrenia. Imaginations turn pathological when the line between facts as we experience them becomes blurred with the fantasy that we create in our minds.

In Southern literature, standard phrases describe how the fragile, white-magnolia female avoids the responsibility of facing life. She "takes to her bed." This means that she uses phrases like, "I'm tired," "exhausted," "I need to rest," followed by holing up in her bedroom, as a tool to get others to serve or wait on her.

Children don't often take to their beds. But they do often "take to their televisions." They use the trance to avoid parents, chores, getting dressed, or going to grandmother's.

We often use FRST to avoid feeling fear, shame, or sadness. We would rather sleep than feel these painful feelings. Although fear, shame, and sadness can resolve into FRST, these emotions rarely help us out of the emotion of FRST. Who wants to wake up to fear, shame, or sadness? Most of us would rather cling to sleep. Why would a child want to leave the television trance only to feel defeated, afraid, or embarrassed?

Positive Consequences of FRST

We have already discussed how rest can nurture our bodies and minds. It is clear that we need to sleep a significant part of every day and relax at least part of the day. After exertion or after being threatened and finding sanctuary, to maintain the quality of our lives we must be able to calm down or self-soothe.

All major religions discuss using faith to combat the fear demons. Indeed, fear can become a force that sabotages instead of protecting us. Bad things happen to good people. Tornadoes, earthquakes, fires, floods, accidents, crimes, and disease can make any one of us a sudden victim. We strive to overcome these ordeals. But often, as we address life's difficulties, we might be unable to make a bad situation better; we can't help but be afraid. Fear fills our bodies with anxiety and tension, and we feel we can do nothing with our emotional energy except be overcome with dread.

We could do something if we knew how and that something is to calm down, go into a trance, relax, rest, and sleep. If we have the skill to relax in the face of adversity, we are combating fear with faith—faith that for this minute we are safe, safe enough to put down our weapons and tools, close our eyes, rest, and renew our bodies and minds.

Rest is often the next—and best—thing for us to do in stressful times. Yet, some of us do not know how to calm down. We therapists must teach those who do not know, how to control their tension. But first, we must learn this skill for ourselves. Inducing the trance in ourselves is a step toward self-soothing. This begins with a reminder that we are safe for the moment, and we can allow ourselves to feel tired.

Feeling tired means that our bodies are breathing quietly, as if we were asleep. Our chest is still, and our bellies move as we breathe. This is called diaphragmatic breathing (Benson, et al., 1975). Once our breathing is quiet and deep, we need to focus our minds on a familiar memory, story, or place that is calming, somewhere we feel safe and confident. Or, we can choose a phrase or sound to repeat over and over that calms us. We can let this imaginary safe place, or safe sound, rock our spirit into a trance. This trance can at least provide rest that possibly will become sleep.

Overusing the trance can create unhealthy consequences. But sometimes this is the best and only defense we have. The child constantly faced with abuse eventually will become dependent on the trance. Soldiers in wartime use the trance to get their minds off war and back to times that they remember fondly. To some this might look like psychosis or delusional thinking, when in fact, the person is using his or her best available survival skill.

Psychologists often use terms like repression and denial to describe the process of pushing fear away with faith, which allows rest and renewal. This skill is not deviant or crazy. It can be the best response to overwhelming stress. Children might discover this skill by themselves and needn't be taught. But when they depend on the trance as their only coping device, this can present a problem.

Our children live in a frightening world. Adults dominate. Children have little power. They don't know how to get what they want. Anger only gets them into trouble, yet they don't want to feel the debilitating effects of fear and sadness. So children choose to "zone out" in front of the TV or stare into space, thinking of nothing or escaping to an imaginary world or an imaginary friend.

A child is practicing self-soothing by repeating familiar behavior, such as fingering a blanket over and over, or asking you to read the same bedtime book for the fifth consecutive night. Repetitive familiar behavior gives children a sense of control and predictability. Before we reprimand them for sucking their thumbs repeatedly or try to interest our children in a different bedtime story because we are bored, remember, repetitive behavior is inherently self-soothing. The familiar makes coping with a trauma much easier.

Fatigue Magnifies

Each emotion has its job and serves a complementary function for the other emotions. Surprise is the emotional clutch or segue. Anger is the emotional defense that protects us from having to feel too much fear, shame, or sadness.

Fatigue, however, if not relieved by sleep, can magnify an emotion beyond reason or normal expectations. Imagine an all-girls slumber party. The girls stay up late. The evening begins with laughter, but as it gets later and the girls get more tired, the giggling becomes constant, and what they are laughing about is not that funny. Or, imagine a policeman who, because he is working two jobs, hasn't had much sleep. He stops a motorist who talks back in a foul tone, and the policeman overreacts in anger. Or, recall being tired and sad at the same time, beginning to cry and having trouble stopping?

For most of us, this tendency for fatigue to amplify our feelings is not a good thing. It can create disproportionate responses to others. People have difficulty understanding such extreme emotional responses. Fatigue can cloud our judgment, allowing emotional impulses to govern behavior, taking us far away from our good sense.

When we are tired and our feelings amplified, others' emotions can become more contagious. We are susceptible to group consensus and less able to think with our own minds and react as individuals.

Groups trying to convince and encourage membership, for example, church youth groups, Werner Erhard Training, and fraternity pledging, often use fatigue to break down defenses to emotions and create shared emotional experiences that help bond the group and encourage self-disclosure and joining. In such circumstances, individuals go along with the group and do and say things that they ordinarily would not.

It's good for us to work up a good sweat, try hard or play hard, become physically worn out, and need rest. Just as our emotions need to flow from one to another, our bodies need to go from one type of activity to another. Our experience of being tired or fatigued tells us that we need to sleep, or at the very least, we need to sit or lie down.

Fatigue becomes a problem when we ignore its signs and continue our work or play. This is especially true for children. Children often are not self-aware enough to take a nap or go to bed. In spite of their yawns or irritability, they want to be part of the activities around them. We must learn to attend to the messages that fatigue sends us so that we can enjoy the success that comes from a daily routine that includes sufficient rest.

Adults use drugs like caffeine or other stimulants so they can continue to work or play, despite the fact that their bodies need rest. Although there is no single standard for how much sleep we require in a day, children usually need more rest than adults.

We must learn to listen to our body's cues telling us that we need rest. Our good sense, emotional balance, character, and reputation might be at stake. Therapists often can help clients best find sanity by referring them to a sleep clinic, because they are chronically sleep deprived.

The Trance, Television, and Children

One thing is clear from research on children and violence: After children watch violent programming, they act more aggressively and are more likely to perpetrate violence themselves. Most often this is explained in terms of modeling theory (Bandura, 1973).

While modeling what we see on television is certainly one plausible explanation, another could be that television is trance-inducing. When in a trance, what we hear and see can have a powerful effect on us. This is the basis of hypnotism. We are easily influenced when we are in a trance (Erickson, Rossi, & Rossi, 1976).

What this means to parents is that they must be careful what children are exposed to when their minds have been given over to the suggestions of an external, trance-inducing force. This might be a stranger with a hypnotic voice and some candy, a popular recorded song, or a children's book that creates frightening images, or, of course, the television.

Only 20% of our nations' families use V-chip technology to prevent children from seeing sex and violence on television. Even parents using the V-chip cannot screen out commercials using sex or provocative, violent action to sell products. And today new trance-inducing video screens offer video games and Internet chat rooms.

While children can derive numerous benefits from television, video games, and the Internet, danger is also present. Parents must be aware of what their children are watching on television, what video games they are playing, and where they go on the Internet. Watching television, playing video games, and surfing the Web are inherently passive activities. Children need to use their bodies and minds to develop creative skills to entertain themselves when they are bored; they should not simply turn on the television and descend into a trance.

The trance creates easy access to children's minds. If we use the trance to teach children, we should assure that they are learning our values. In our role as therapists, we can encourage clients to protect their children from dangerous trance inductions. Here are points to discuss with clients:

- read to your children;
- select appropriate films that both you and your children can attend. Talk with them about what they see;
- limit television viewing to 1 hour a day. Set aside 2 or 3 days a week of "no-television days;"
- plan family activities during times when you once watched TV. Go out for ice cream after supper. Read a book aloud together, have family game night, go for a walk in the neighborhood;
- encourage your children to pursue a hobby; make drawing materials, basketball goals, and bicycles available so that your children can learn to entertain themselves.

Therapists have children, too, and should consider applying this advice to their children.

The Trance Metaphor and Therapists

How do art, literature, and film profoundly affect the human psyche? The answer is that somehow these media put us in a trance.

In the media-induced trance, we connect with our own emotions, memories, and imaginations. While in this state, we combine these to create a transformative human experience. When our imaginations begin to transport us from our current experience, we are in a trance. The trance creates access to our past, present, and imagined future; our hurts, fears, and joys.

Art can give us a real experience that was completely imagined. Through the trance, art can change our souls.

Carkhuff's famous text (1969), training therapists in empathic listening, proposes five levels of empathy. Level three is an accurate reflection of the client's feelings. Level four adds a dimension of meaning that accurately reflects the client's feelings and extends and deepens them. Level five is similar to level four, except that the listener's response adds even greater depth and meaning that accurately resonates with the client's experiences.

Larry Weitz, my professor in an introductory counseling practicum, called level five "listening metaphorically." He said only master therapists could do this. When one is able to listen to another and form images and concrete imaginary visions of the client's experiences, the therapist strengthens the therapeutic alliance and deepens the therapist's access to the client. This kind of empathy gives the client a sense of safety and trust, allowing the therapist to participate more effectively with the client in change and growth.

I contend that reflecting metaphorically in this way creates a partial trance. It engages the client's imagination with an image—an image like, "That sounds like how it would feel to climb a sheer cliff." Or, "You sound as happy as a hog in a corn patch." Or, "That must be like trying to swim a mile with boots on."

Milton Erickson, the father of modern hypnosis, paradoxical intervention, and neurolinguistic programming, points to metaphors as the central device in hypnotic induction. Images from memories or fantasy surely can initiate the trance. At times, therapists deliberately use the trance to help clients stop smoking, manage pain, or build self-esteem and self-respect.

Some have wrongly used the trance as a memory-retrieval device, thus creating memories, instead of discovering them. For us, the point of this malpractice is that the trance is profoundly powerful. Access to the trance in a client can give the therapist an amazing amount of influence.

Just as clients need to be careful what their children are exposed to in a trance, therapists must also be careful with how we use metaphors and the trance. In the best of circumstances, we therapists can use the trance, not to invent new pain for our clients, but to facilitate growth and insight.

Eye movement desensitization and reprocessing (EMDR) is a new form of therapy that has proved surprisingly effective. The therapist creates a repetitive shift of attention in the client, using the eyes, hearing, or tactile sensation. It is believed that this rapid shifting of attention activates the REM sleep mechanism while the client is awake, creating a simulated trance state.

In sleep, it is believed that REM brain activity stimulates the neocortex to make sense of the vivid memories stored in the hippocampus. The neocortex creates a reasonable narrative from these memories that helps us make meaning, thus creating closure that resolves the threats created by these events. Rapidly shifting attention in this way modulates the release of acetylcholine in the brain. This inhibits the startle response from overwhelming the neocortex's processing of the strong memories and allows the neocortex to complete the work of meaning-making so that internal peace can be made with these events.

When the therapist induces this trance in a client, the client can process painful memories more effectively. This could be the reason why this procedure is so effective with clients suffering from post-traumatic stress.[11]

Teaching Self-Soothing Skills

When we want to soothe ourselves, the CALMS ritual is very useful. The actor's dead-face routine is an alternative (see chapter 6.) We must help clients reduce stimuli and distract their minds from their current circumstance. Relaxation tapes are excellent resources. But clients often can draw on their own resources.

Consider the function of counting sheep to help us sleep. This is certainly a boring activity. One student I observed used his chemistry text to help him sleep. As soon as he opened it, his eyes became heavy. Sex can be an excellent precursor to sleep, as is a warm bath or hot milk. Familiar and repetitive rituals are soothing as well.

In the twenty-first century, every therapist should have his or her own system of teaching clients this skill. There is little more to add than to emphasize the importance of self-soothing as an emotionally healing tool (see chapter 6).

Resolving FRST

Any emotion will resolve FRST. Awaking is a general arousal characterized by interest/excitement/desire. "I've got to go to the bathroom" is a desire that wakes me in the morning. My cat sleeps through the night without a sound, but at 6 a.m. she wakes with loud and persistent meowing, signaling her interest in food.

Shame, fear, sadness, and *anger* are not pleasant emotions to wake up to. *Surprise* can be abrupt. *Disgust* is certainly an essential emotion to our survival (e.g., waking disgusted to a smelly, smoke-filled room can save our lives in a fire). *Joy* would be a wonderful emotion to wake up to. But most of the time, joy comes after interest provoked an arousal toward a goal. When the goal is achieved, joy is the result.

Other emotions have paths that take two or three emotions to resolve. For fatigue, only one emotion is necessary, and that emotion is *interest*. Interest arouses us and puts us back into a new emotional flow.

Fatigue teaches an important lesson relevant to all emotions. Clearly, we need to relax and rest until we have had enough rest. The same applies to sadness, fear, joy, and so forth. We should not awake from one emotion until we have expressed as much of it as we feel necessary.

We often stop feeling sad prematurely and, for example, paste a smile on our faces when we actually have a great deal more sadness to express. A balance exists with every emotion. We all hope to find that place in expressing our feelings, somewhere between not enough and too much.

We frequently have difficulty breaking out of a trance and letting go of a delusion. The trance is often more pleasant than reality. In fact, that is the point of the trance: to anesthetize us from the fears that we can do nothing about. The problem with the trance is that it can paralyze us so that we do nothing when, in reality, it would be useful for us to act. Most of us cannot admit that we are in a trance. But for the lucky few who can, the following is a helpful process that will break them free from the trance and ground them in the present reality. We will use **AWAKE** as our acronym.

 Step 1: **A**rouse yourself—give yourself the same energy you would have if you were suddenly startled. Look around you.

 Step 2: **W**here, **W**hat, **W**hy and Ho**w**—use these four questions to orient yourself to the present. Where are you? What is really happening? Why are you here now? How did you get here?

 Step 3: **A**sk yourself what feeling you were using the trance to avoid. Often it is fear or sadness, or shame, or longing. Claim that feeling and feel it. Face the reality that you have used the trance to avoid.

 Step 4: **K**now what others see. Test reality by asking trusted friends what they see. Confirm your sense of reality by using your community of friends and family. We all distort reality and fall into trances. We sometimes need help in seeing reality as it is.

 Step 5: **E**ngage life again without the trance. Be in the present. Work to change what you need to change so that you won't need to avoid reality with a trance.

Summary and Conclusion

My conversation with Marietta continued. As you might recall, I was in pretty deep. Our last words were from Marietta: "Am I so awful that you have to run away from me?" My reply was "No, of course not. What are you saying?"

Marietta continued, "I'm saying that when we are together alone on a vacation, I don't feel very loved or important. If we go with other couples or in a group, you don't write, and you are very responsive to our travel companions."

"You tell me not to take a writing project along because it is rude, and I don't," I said.

"Well, it is rude. It's rude to me, too. I guess I don't count."

"Of course you count. I didn't realize what I was doing to you till now. It is rude. I'm ashamed I didn't see this before. The thing that I'm most interested in is being with you on vacation. That's part of the reason we take vacations, because it is good for us to get away together. I will quit writing right now."

"You don't have to do that."

"Oh, yes I do, and you know it. Thanks for waking me up out of my trance. This gives us an opportunity to really be together."

For the rest of the vacation I used the AWAKE ritual every day to keep me connected to what was really important to me. And that was Marietta. It helped.

CHAPTER 13

Disgust/Contempt
The Discerning Emotion

Disgust/Contempt Defined

Disgust for our purposes is combined with contempt. The survival function of these two emotions is to avoid poison or contamination. This could be from eating or touching, or from emotional poison or social contamination. The social function of these emotions is basically offensive and intended to harm or reject. The human object of these emotions is meant to feel shame and be repelled.

Darwin defined disgust as "something revolting, primarily in relation to the sense of taste ... and, secondarily, to anything that causes a similar feeling through the sense of smell, touch, or eyesight" (1872, p. 65, p. 253). Tomkins (1963) used similar words but placed more emphasis on interpersonal intimacy. According to Tomkins, disgust is "recruited to defend the self against psychic incorporation or any increase in intimacy with a repellant object" (ibid., p. 233).

The survival function of disgust/contempt is to protect the body from poison, disease, or infection. It can be elicited by food; body products; and associations with sex, death, or hygiene. Evolution in humans has expanded disgust from the biological functions to include moral and social functions. It serves to protect the soul and the social order, as well as the body. Strangers, people different from us, those considered undesirable, and moral offenses can also elicit disgust/contempt.

As we evolved, so did disgust. What is disgusting varied according to the culture, the family, and the person.

Douglas (1966) implied that disgust is our reaction to something out of bounds or in the wrong place. Though disgust has made every list of emotions, it is not present in monkeys. It appears to be a distinguishing feature of the human species (Chevalier-Skolnikoff, 1973).

The biological purpose of disgust/contempt is to discriminate among tastes. This emotion protects us from what we judge to be a source of contamination, disease, or poison. It warns us to get away from, not eat, keep a clean kitchen, and touch with a stick rather than with our hands. While the evolutionary base of disgust/contempt centers on food, we use it symbolically to express our negative judgment and rejection of things, people and behavior we disapprove of.

Many of us can remember a time when we saw our beloved with another person and felt sick to our stomach with disgust. Our face mimics the expression that automatically comes with nausea. Our nose wrinkles as we raise our upper lip; our lower lip and tongue protrude. That is the facial expression of disgust.

We all recognize the facial expression that comes with being lied to or cheated. Our natural response is contempt. Our nose goes up in the air as if we were withdrawing from an offending odor; one corner of our mouth is raised, while the other is lowered. This expression is called the sneer of contempt. For our purposes, we will consider these emotions as one.

Clinical Case Study

I was seeing Jerry and Liz. They had been on the brink of divorce, but they were backing away a bit and getting along better. In one session, Jerry recounted his teenage school years.

"Ever since you told us about this Gottman fellow and his research showing that marriages were headed for divorce when couples' fights included shaming, humiliating, sarcastic remarks, I began to notice how often I used mean words with Liz," Jerry explained. "I think it was something I started as a kid, like you told us when you said eighth graders overused disgust. You said disgust is most often practiced by teenagers. I had never thought about practicing disgust. You said it had a purpose in teaching us who we are, what we do like and do not. I picked up on disgust as a teen, and I guess I never quit using it.

"I remember I had a great seventh grade math teacher, Mr. Stanford. He was the first teacher who called us by our last names only. It was 'Aldridge, sit down, shut up, or get out,' or 'Aldridge, get your head out of the gutter and come to the board and work this problem.'"

"Mr. Stanford defined cynicism and sarcasm. He made us laugh. We loved him—except when we were the butt of his joke—even then, it wasn't too bad, because we all had our turn.

"My friends and I became accomplished at using our disgust to humiliate others. We joked about a girl who was overweight. We tormented a boy whose face was disfigured with acne. We ridiculed a girl plagued by eczema.

"On the first day of football practice one year, Jack Townsend came out for football for the first time. His father had died when he was a boy, and his mother and grandmother were raising him. He had never seen a naked body other than his own. When he got in the shower with all the other naked boys, Jack had an erection. From that day forward, my homophobic friends and I called him 'queer Townsend.' I guess I thought that was fun. I guess I never grew out of playing with disgust."

The Neurology of Disgust/Contempt

Like other negative emotions, disgust/contempt is associated with the right frontal area (Davidson, 1992), thus confirming its late evolution in the brain. The basal ganglia appears to be the center of disgust/contempt in the brain (Sprengelmeyer, et al., 1997).

Research has yet to define disgust circuitry in the brain. I would speculate that there would be a link to the amygdala, since disgust can stimulate the brain's vigilance system. Since disgust can turn off appetites and initiate withdrawal from intimacy, it appears likely that the septal area of the brain participates in the disgust/contempt response, as well as the thalamocingulate circuit (Davidson, 1992).

I have found little written about the neurohormones associated with disgust. Disgust/contempt implicitly entitles a person to judge; that would associate it, therefore, with ego-strength and high levels of serotonin (5-H7). As disgust turns off sexual interest, it is likely to be negatively correlated with amounts of gonadtropin-releasing hormone (GnRH). Monoamine oxidase (MAO) also might play a role.

The endorphins that provide opiates associated with pleasure are likely negatively associated with disgust. Cholecystokinin (CCK) is associated with fear and appetite regulation. One could speculate that disgust would be associated positively with this neurohormone.

The Physiology of Disgust/Contempt

The primary physiological change that is associated with disgust/contempt is nausea (Darwin, 1965). Increased salivation is also associated with nausea (and hence disgust) (Miller, 1997).

Just as there is little research on neurohormones of disgust/contempt, little is known about the physiology of disgust/contempt. In spite of a large literature devoted to the search for physiological signatures of different emotions, I know of no experimental studies on the relationship of disgust/contempt to nausea or salivation. Rather, the research on the physiological side of disgust/contempt has been limited to the standard set of autonomic responses explored by psychophysiologists.

In this limited arena, it appears that disgust/contempt is associated with a parasympathetic nervous system response, whereas fear and anger are associated with a predominantly sympathetic nervous system (Levenson, Ekman, & Friesen, 1990; Levenson, 1992).

The Intelligence of Disgust/Contempt

I would speculate that disgust/contempt is highly intelligent. Located in the highly evolved front of the brain (Davidson, 1992), it is one of the last emotions to evolve in humans. To be disgusted or contemptuous, we must discriminate, or logically evaluate the source of the distaste or nausea. We need our intellect to make the discriminations and judgments that are part of disgust/contempt.

The Negative Consequences of Disgust/Contempt

Izard (1972) first conceptualized what he called the "hostility triad" of emotions. He identified these as contempt, anger, and disgust. These three emotions when viewed by an uninterested observer are the three most unattractive emotions. Most of us are repelled by the person expressing these feelings. That is their point, of course, to push away or intimidate someone into leaving and submitting. But in addition to frightening and shaming their object, these emotions repel the observer as well.

Disgust/contempt is the basis of all kinds of discrimination and prejudice. These emotions entitled Hitler to attempt to eliminate the Jews, and Americans to exterminate Indians or hold slaves. It is the basis of wars and social hatred.

Disgust/contempt also can be linked to obsessive-compulsive disorder. When we suffer from this illness, we are obsessed with what we believe to be disgusting, and we use ritualistic behaviors to protect ourselves from contact with things such as repeated hand washing; turning the light switch on and off five times to be sure nothing has changed in the room; ritualistic vomiting by bulimic clients.

Disgust/contempt tends to give permission to anger, thus releasing behavior motivated by our least intelligent emotion. This can result in inappropriate behavior and poor judgment.

Disgust/contempt of others can be a product of repressed self-disgust. This intense rejection of the self can produce a multitude of ill-advised, mean, self-destructive, and pathological behaviors.

The Positive Consequences of Disgust/Contempt

If I have a least favorite emotion, this is it. It is difficult for me to consider disgust as a valuable emotional tool. I would rather ignore it, hoping that it would go away. But that doesn't square with the thesis of this book: all emotions serve an important adaptive function. Our job is to use disgust/contempt as a tool for good purposes and be careful not to get stuck in it, or to avoid feeling it (or any of our feelings).

The function of disgust/contempt in the development of a self is that it teaches us right from wrong and good from bad, and distinguishes justice from injustice and human kindness from evil. Disgust/contempt has many parallels in how religion often is regarded in our culture. Religion is criticized as being the basis of wars, religious hatred, and intolerance. Yes, of course, this is true, just as it is true about disgust/contempt. But religion is also responsible for teaching love, compassion, kindness, and tolerance. This too is true about disgust/contempt. It can be a force for good as well as bad. Its effect depends on how we use it.

On the political right, Bill Bennett wrote a book called *The Death of Outrage* (1998), advocating that we should be intolerant, disgusted by, and contemptuous of certain behavior displayed by President Clinton. From a leftist point of view, Bennett's judgment is termed "sexual McCarthyism," or evil and dangerous witch-hunting intolerance.

The national debate on the matter can be compared on a small scale with the dilemma these emotions present us. We want to have standards and know right from wrong. We want to have disgust and contempt for dangerous drugs; casual, uncommitted, and unprotected sex; and unlawful behavior. We want to drive safely and wear a seat belt. We want to condemn stealing or raping. We want to be disgusted when classmates cheat on tests. We want to value the truth. The likes and dislikes that come from disgust/contempt are the basis of society's values.

Disgust/contempt is the emotion of discernment and judgment. We want to have taste—in behavior, color and design, music and harmony. It creates the basis for deciding what we like and what we do not. While interest/excitement represents the emotion that says what we like and are attracted to, disgust/contempt represents the emotion we express when things repulse us. What would we be without this emotion? We would be wishy-washy people with no standards and no limits on behavior. We need likes and dislikes; else we have no values. There is no definition of the self without disgust/contempt.

The Role of Parents in Guiding Children through Disgust/Contempt

No one teaches disgust and contempt to children. It is a reflexive response to what they put in their mouths. Yet at some point, children transfer from their mouths to their minds the symbolic representation of disgust/contempt. So disgust/contempt becomes associated with all dislikes. Parents must help their children make appropriate social discriminations about what is and should be considered disgusting and contemptuous and what should not.

Many of us have taught our children that people with skin color different from ours are worthy of disgust/contempt. This is a clear abuse of parental authority and perpetuates evil and prejudice. But parents are correct in passing on certain prejudices to their children. Some parents are offended by smoking in general and by smoking in crowded places in particular. Some parents are repulsed by pornography and the misogyny that is implicit in it. Some parents are contemptuous of lies and value truth-telling.

As the primary socializing agent of our children, we pass on our values to them. In *The Death of Outrage*, Bennett asserts that we are failing to teach our children values. We are afraid of making moral judgments, even though our civilization, the safety and security of our children and families, and our economy and justice system depend on the making of moral judgments and the passing of values from one generation to the next.

This is the theme of the Old Testament prophets, calling the Israelites back to their fundamental values of right and wrong. The prophets' claim was that Israel would become lost without commitment to God's law, without disgust and contempt for behavior that breaks those laws.

But when you read the preceding paragraph, doesn't it make you a bit nervous? Don't you naturally ask, who are we to judge and condemn others? How do we know what's right for someone else? We can't speak for God, can we?

Certainly, as therapists, we must restrain ourselves from imposing our values on our clients. Our job is to help clients discover their values, their own disgust. As parents, we have a responsibility to model healthy values to our children. Parents have influence over their children's choices. Children will value what their parents value. Parents' words won't matter nearly as much as their behavior. Children likely will smoke if their parents do. They likely will divorce if their parents have. They likely will study hard if their parents did and become good parents if their parents were.

None of us has the right to condemn other people to hell or to social purgatory. But we all have the right to condemn behavior that we find disgusting. And we have the responsibility to explain to our children why we have contempt for this behavior.

The Role of the Therapist

Nathanson (1992) states that clients whose mothers have used the emotion of disgust/contempt as their primary socializing tool with their child seem to be unable to form a lasting primary relationship. There is obviously much psychic pain that this emotion can sow. But what can we therapists do about it?

Should we have contempt for these mothers who have disgust for their children? "Yes," is the answer of some therapists. Should we have contempt for the fathers who didn't protect their children from their contemptuous mothers? "Yes," is the answer of other therapists.

A systems-trained therapist would point out that these emotional behavior patterns are passed from one generation to the next. If we are trying to find an object for our contempt and a person to blame, in what generation will we land?

Our primary job is similar to a parent's job:

1. Understand, have compassion, see that we are all alike. We all feel;
2. Help our clients have compassion for their parents. Focus the contempt on the behavior, which probably is disgusting, and help the client have compassion for their parents who acted in this disgusting way;
3. Help them have compassion for themselves, trapped by generations of this behavior. Encourage them to take on the species' task of being an improvement on what went before. We should all be an improvement on the generation that preceded. But probably the generations following us will still have work to do. And that is the way it has been and the way it will be for some time.

That speaks to the person who is the victim of their disgust. But what are we therapists to do when our clients behave in ways that disgust us? One answer is don't work with them. If we are disgusted by smoking in our office and a client states that she cannot refrain from smoking for an hour, refer her. If you are recently divorced because your mate had an extramarital affair (and you still feel betrayed and contemptuous of your ex-spouse) and a client comes to you in the midst of an affair, don't see that individual, refer her.

These are easy answers. What do we do when clients use the "N" word, tell a racist or sexist joke, or abuse their wives? Some of these are things that some of us might choose to ignore. Others, like child abuse, we are required by law not to ignore. Generally, our job is to help clients like these see that this behavior does not define them, that it comes as a defense against their fears or shame. It is something that they did. We should oppose them continuing in these disgusting behaviors. But we should tell them that we believe they can do better and give them the emotional skills they need in order to grow and change their disgusting, destructive, habitual response patterns.

Disgust/Contempt and Self-Esteem

Too often, we gain pride and self-esteem at the expense of others. We use disgust/contempt emotions to elevate us to a superior, better-than position.

Remember when you were a child and one of your peers blew her nose in her hands (perhaps because she couldn't afford tissue or a handkerchief?) She became the butt of class jokes. Other children were proud and felt good that they were not like her. Everything she did became synonymous with disgust/contempt. All the other children boosted their self-esteem at the expense of this girl.

Adults do the same thing with cars, houses, degrees, and money. We find ways to amass self-esteem by honoring people who have certain things or qualities, while having contempt for those who do not. This is false self-esteem. It depends on things outside us, rather than on things inside us.

Authentic self-esteem comes from our battles with ourselves. We all want to have sex with a good-looking movie star. We all want all the money that is in the bank. We all are tempted, and we all struggle with our temptations. We all get tired and want to give in to our impulses.

How do we really judge ourselves? Do we judge ourselves by the clothes we wear, the car we drive, or the house we live in? Others might, but most of us evaluate ourselves by how we control our own behavior. Are we faithful to our commitments? Do we bend the truth to suit our purposes? Do we know what our best effort is, and do we give it? Do we do what is right or what feels good? How we answer these questions has much more to do with our self-esteem than the car we drive.

Disgust/contempt applied to our behavior can be useful in helping us develop the self-discipline and self-control that is essential to self-esteem. If we apply our values to ourselves, first, before we judge others, we are likely to develop these qualities. Of course, you want to protect your clients from the shame of being disgusted with the essence of their souls. But you do hope that they feel disgusted with their lies, with not keeping a promise, or with not giving their best effort.

Shame and self-disgust/contempt are closely related. The distinction between these two emotions is the audience. The audience for our healthy shame is our community. Shame helps us reweave our torn social fabric. It motivates us to make amends. It brings confession, contrition, apology, and behavior aimed at healing the wounds we caused in others.

The audience for self-disgust/contempt is the self, not the community. The goal is not to make amends as much as it is to protect, improve, and control the self. These are worthy goals when the object of self-disgust/contempt is changing behavior, but it is pathological when disgust/contempt is aimed at our souls.

Treating Self-Disgust

We've all seen children display their self-contempt in a temper-tantrum. There is the child playing baseball who strikes out at home plate and in disgust bangs her own head with her bat; or the child who lies on the ground slamming her fists into the dirt because she failed to complete a cartwheel correctly.

We adults can behave in similar ways. A career can collapse, and, at midlife, we can go fishing and let our spouses pick up the pieces. Children can grow up and leave home—sometimes in a fit of temper, or possibly without saying anything. When they leave, we might just take to our bedroom, watch CNN or the soaps, and emerge only to go to the grocery store. We might feel like failures, and be disgusted with ourselves.

We want children to use self-disgust/contempt to prevent them from behaving badly or challenge and spur them on toward improvement. But when clients indulge in a self-destructive tantrum of self-directed disgust and we, as therapists, watch passively, we are accepting this behavior and endorsing self-hatred.

Yes, it is a good thing for us and our clients to be our own authorities, have standards, and display disgust for our behavior when we don't try or don't face reality. But part of self-discipline and self-control involves learning to manage our feelings. Excessive self-anger or disgust/contempt can lead to either too much emotional intensity or to hopelessness and giving up. Being self-critical is one thing, but engaging in self-hatred or a self-directed temper-tantrum creates a loss of confidence and takes away our focus and concentration, diverting it into emotional theater rather than effective performance.

As therapists, we should encourage clients not to give up. A mistake is just a mistake. While it is fine to be self-critical of our efforts, it is never fair to ourselves or to others to be excessively critical of results. We therapists should teach clients that positive results come with practice, self-discipline, and emotional self-control.

We should help clients remember that they will only do their best if they like and respect themselves, regardless of how things turn out. We can believe messages we tell ourselves when we are indulging in a self-disgust temper-tantrum. These are mostly lies, but we have no one inside our heads to defend us. Clients will recognize them as lies. It is our job to point out these unnecessary self-flagellations.

When these feelings dominate our emotional landscape, we can become hypercritical of ourselves and others. We become terrified of contamination by objects that repulse us. We might defend ourselves from the germs of the world by washing our hands ten times a day. Or, we might develop magical rituals to ward off calamitous events, such as avoiding stepping on cracks in the sidewalk or lifting our feet when our car crosses railroad tracks.

Some of us do not outgrow these superstitious rituals and develop bizarre myths. We can come to believe that danger will befall us if we don't repeat our obsessive rituals or if our vigilance fails and we somehow step on a crack. Therapists might find they are ineffective at helping these clients return to reality. Clients frequently hide their bizarre behaviors and thoughts from their therapists. And when we therapists try to present reality to our clients, they might refuse to be convinced.

This is especially evident in the anorexic girl who is starving herself because she is disgusted by her body, which she perceives as fat. Her parents, teachers, doctors, and therapists can tell her that her 5-foot frame with its 70 pounds needs more weight and that she is dying. But these words have little impact on her mind's-eye view of her body.

Two things are helpful to such hypersensitive and self-critical clients. One is the drug fluoxetine, otherwise known as Prozac. This drug is a member of a family of drugs (SSRIs) that have been useful to clients who seem to be stuck in obsessive worry, centering on feelings of disgust/contempt.

A second way is for therapists to help these clients understand the feelings beneath their self-disgust. Most of the time their obsessive behaviors cover feelings of fear and shame. We can help our clients become aware of their fears and face them, using their fears to make plans and proceeding toward self-fulfilling goals (see chapter 6).

We can help clients transform their shame into pride (see chapter 10). We should understand that this compulsive behavior might be inherited, not simply learned, and that patience and love are the best resources available in coping with clients who seemingly cannot liberate themselves from self-disgust. Don't abandon the field until clients learn for themselves that they are worthy and valuable. Liking themselves, having a healthy narcissism is genetic too. The therapist's job is to help our clients rediscover this.

The Passive/Unassertive Client

Some of us—and our clients—do not use the emotions of disgust/contempt. If we are seeing clients who were easily influenced to do what they feel is wrong, we must be careful not to join them in their self-disgust. If we do, we can become a central figure in a new drama titled, "Judgmental Therapist/Victim Client."

Instead, we should allow clients to discover the natural consequences of their behavior. Remember, their pain is their best teacher, not our disapproval, and they will feel their pain if we don't distract them. Our job is to help them milk their pain for all the wisdom it can give them; help them use their disgust to define their personal likes and dislikes; and help them develop their use of disgust as a way to protect themselves from the destructive behavior that will inevitably bring shame with it.

As much as possible, therapists must keep their own anger and personal judgments out of our clients' way. Clients need an unobstructed view of their personal experience as they use disgust to protect themselves and develop their personal identity.

Resolving Disgust/Contempt

What best resolves disgust/contempt?

Anger usually multiplies and adds to disgust/contempt. It rarely diminishes it. *Fear* might repress disgust. But it only keeps it below the surface and can transform external disgust into self-disgust. The energy that comes from the union of anger and disgust can bring the joy of victory. But this joy will only institutionalize disgust and entitle us to continue feeling it. *Joy* and disgust together become ridicule. Joy is rarely a healthy resolve for disgust.

Shame is the emotion most closely associated with disgust. It is the emotion disgust attempts to make its object feel (and usually that is someone else). But it works the other way as well. If we feel disgust/contempt and find out we are wrong or we lose and are vanquished by our foes, shame will resolve our disgust/contempt. This is not a pleasant outcome.

Sadness is a leveling emotion, and it will resolve disgust, reminding us that we are all losing somehow. After all, life is tragic.

Shame and sadness are effective resolves for disgust, but the best resolution to disgust is surprise followed by interest. Disgust/contempt gives us certainty and confidence that right is with us. When we recruit *surprise* or when someone (perhaps a therapist) invites us into the not-knowing, wonder place, it takes away this certainty. If surprise is followed by the energy that comes from interest, the combination of surprise and interest creates curiosity. This leads to research and study, which we hope will bring new information. Information will solidify good values or diminish our disgust.

One day I was asked to observe child-caregiver interaction at a local kindergarten. I observed the following interchange between Leotha, an African American daycare worker, and Bobby, a 4-year-old boy.

"My uncle says black people are dirty, and they smell," Bobby said. "He said if I touch you or if you touch me, I will get all dirty and smelly."

It was clear to me that Bobby was confused. Leotha was being attentive and kind to Bobby. He obviously wanted her attention, but he was ambivalent.

"I'm not dirty," Leotha said. "If you touch me, you won't get dirty. Do you want to touch me and see?"

Bobby was reluctant.

"Touch my hand," she said.

"OK," Bobby agreed. And he touched the palm of her hand.

"Did you get dirty when you touched my hand?"

"But that part of you is white. It's not as black as the rest of you."

"Touch my arm."

And Bobby did.

"Did your fingers get dirty?" she asked.

"No, they are not dirty," Bobby said, relieved.

"Smell my wrist if you want, Bobby," and Bobby sniffed her wrist and forearm.

"Do I smell?"

"No, well, yes. You smell like Ivory soap."

She smelled Bobby's arm. "And you smell like Dial soap."

"So Uncle Carl is wrong?" he asked.

"Well, I think so."

"Is Uncle Carl wrong about other black people?"

"Everybody is different. You are white, and sometimes you are dirty and you smell. If your mother didn't bathe you, you would stay smelly and dirty. Some black people are smelly and dirty sometimes, just like some white people. Find out for yourself. Don't judge people by what somebody else says."

Leotha didn't respond to Bobby's disgust with her own version of disgust for Bobby's prejudice. Disgust returned is the most often used reflexive response, disgust triggering disgust, triggering disgust, ad infinitum. This is what is happening in the Middle East, Northern Ireland, and Bosnia and on many playgrounds in America, as one race or religion is pitted against another.

Instead, Leotha resisted her impulse to respond in kind and had compassion for Bobby's ignorance and the difficult position Bobby was in. She understood that Bobby was caught between his urge to like Leotha and loyalty to his uncle's prejudice. Out of compassion, she offered her skin to touch and her body to smell, giving Bobby his own experience that he could use. If he was in fact disgusted, he confirmed his uncle's beliefs. If he was not, he could begin to liberate himself from prejudice.

Leotha resolved Bobby's disgust by inviting him to wonder and then pursue his question with interest, until he had his own experience that he could use to make his own judgment. Leotha was a great therapist. She gave Bobby a chance to form his identity with his own experience, and Bobby accepted her invitation.

If you have a client who overuses disgust, following is a ritual that will help that individual resolve disgust into tolerance and respect, as Leotha helped Bobby. The acronym is **LIMIT**.

 Step 1: Look to discover your personal moral space. Define the values that you use to judge yourself and to judge the behaviors that you want to be a part of and with which you wish to be associated. Enthusiastically express these values and your personal likes and dislikes that you use to judge your own behavior.

 Step 2: Isolate yourself in your role. Define your role in the setting. Are you a member, guest, observer, active participant, initiator, facilitator, teacher, student, leader, owner? Once your role is

clearly defined, express the opinions that your role requires, make the judgments that you are responsible to make in your role, and no more.

 Step 3: <u>M</u>ake appropriate boundaries. Where do you belong? Is it your place to say something? Decide where the social lines should be drawn. It is always your place to speak about yourself and how you feel. It is always your place to decide how you will behave. Usually you are out of bounds when you try to control another or when you make judgments for or about another person. But you are where you belong when you evaluate yourself and your own behavior.

 Step 4: <u>I</u>mpress on yourself and others that you will not talk about a person who is not present. Make it clear to yourself and others that you will repeat what you say about another to that person. Limit yourself to conversation about people present or about things of interest to people present. Avoid gossip and triangular communication.

 Step 5: <u>T</u>olerate opinions and behavior of others that do not require your participation. Offer opinions when asked. Avoid volunteering your random, unconsidered judgment. Understand that others may have different feelings and opinions, because they serve different roles and have had different experiences. Perhaps you can learn from them.

Summary and Conclusion

Remember Liz and Jerry? Jerry had said, "I guess I never grew out of playing with disgust."

"And it hurt me. I didn't think it was funny," Liz responded. "Though I didn't realize it, I guess I developed disgust as my defense against yours. When we had conflicts, things began to get out of hand. They were so bad I wanted to kill you sometimes. We've been practicing this LIMIT ritual, and now we don't use disgust so much. I don't see any reason for that emotion," she added.

"I tend to agree with you," I said, "though sometimes disgust is useful in a crisis. Surgeons need to have a strong feeling of disgust for mistakes in the operating room. Generals need to have a strong feeling of disgust for any decision that might unnecessarily risk the lives of their troops. Quarterbacks need disgust for bad play calling."

"Yet, I wonder if surgeons, generals, and quarterbacks make good husbands?" Liz said. "I'm married to a CEO who used to be a quarterback. Perhaps disgust works well for Jerry at work, but it has not been a good thing in our marriage, or for the children. It's not only words; it's tone of voice."

"I think I see that now," Jerry said. "I think my family has been a victim of my critical successes in my work. Having high standards has been good for my career, but I don't want to create so much pain in my family. I've been using this LIMIT ritual. It has helped me take more time making decisions, slow down my judgments, stay where I belong. I'm not so decisive or opinionated in my work, but I think my colleagues are less intimidated by me. I know my children are. And I hope Liz finds it easier to be married to me."

CHAPTER **14**

Empathy/Compassion/Tending
The Emotional Master Key

Unlocking a New Door

As I began research for this book, I did not intend to mention empathy/compassion/tending. I knew that empathy is magic, it gives the empathizing person self-esteem, and often helps the receiver of compassion bear the burden more easily. What I didn't know was how it works in the brain, or how important a role it fills in our emotional wiring.

I had been influenced by social scientists who use the term "perspective-taking" as a synonym for empathy/compassion/tending. Those using this term frequently suggest that this is a difficult task for many of us, that is, taking the perspective of another. Implicitly the users of the term perspective-taking suggest that empathy is a logical decision that we choose to make or not. I also thought, as they suggest, that empathy is a logical, cognitive, intellectual process—that we look at the other person, identify what that individual feels, put that same emotion on our face and in our minds, reflect it back to that person, showing that we understand and feel the same way. I believed that empathy or compassion was something we choose to express. I thought it was a product of an intellectual process.

My literature search taught me differently. I learned that we use the same brain circuitry to identify an emotion that other people feel and the same brain circuits to express that emotion ourselves. The reception and the awareness of what other people feel comes from the centers in our brains where we experience these same feelings. Thus, we cannot recognize what another person feels without first feeling that feeling ourselves. When clients with brain lesions in the joy-brain circuitry see others feeling joy, they can't

217

recognize the feeling as joy. The same is true with emotions such as fear, anger, and shame (Batson, et al., 1991).

There are neurohormones and brain circuits that support empathy, but these neurochemicals and brain circuits are not the seat of empathy. There is no one place for that. Empathy begins when we see emotion in other people. The same part of their brain that expresses the emotion is stimulated in our brain. We know what they feel because we are now feeling it, too. The neurostructures that support mating, bonding, attachment, and so forth are engaged when we want to tend to someone. If not, we just note, "Oh, that's what they are feeling," and then turn our attention elsewhere. If we do want to nurture someone, the nurturing brain structures and chemicals kick in, and we open up ourselves to feel their feelings more intensely. It is important to emphasize that the basic neurostructures of empathy come from a species instinct to feel with others before we are aware of what they are feeling.

In a normal brain, empathy is a built-in reflex. Feelings are naturally contagious. Remember a time when you were watching a friend talk on the phone? Assume for the moment that nothing in her current setting is a stimulus for the emotion that she expresses, as she and her friend talk. And yet, you witness emotions pouring into her face and voice. She hangs up, and suddenly she addresses you with no emotion at all or in a completely different emotional tone. Where did that phone conversation emotion come from? Why was she feeling it? Where did it go?

Consider a TV commercial that depicts an audience in a movie theater. We see two people, presumably on a date, with a bag of popcorn in one hand and a soft drink in the armchair cup holder. Their faces are filled with emotion, fear one second, anger the next, then sadness, turning into joy. Yet, there is nothing happening in the theater. They are sitting passively among an audience of other passive viewers, staring at a movie screen. No danger, no hurt, no achievement. How could they feel these intense emotions? Where did their feelings come from?

Could the answer to these questions be the answer to why, in Bandura's research, children act out violent behavior after watching violence on television? We know emotions are contagious. Considerable research about the contagion of depression exists (Joiner, 1994). But where does the anger in an angry mob originate? Or the jubilation that can take over a city whose team wins the World Series?

Clinical Case Study

I saw Ann and Harold as a couple. They had been having trouble communicating. Neither of them knew how to listen. They both felt misunderstood and unloved. After working with me for 6 months, they were much better.

"Ann and I had just returned from vacation," Harold said. "We carried in the bags and began unpacking. I finished before Ann and started unloading the answering machine. There were 21 messages, most of which were hang-ups. As I got to message number 19, I heard a familiar voice, that of Ann's cousin, Ralph Singer. His father, Ann's uncle, had died the day before.

"Ann listened intently as I had the machine repeat the message to her. After the message finished, she handed the phone to me and went to the window and stared out. I knew she was sad. I walked behind her and put my arm around her. She looked at me, and I could see the tears brimming in her eyes. Tears filled mine as well. She put her head on my shoulder, and we looked out the window together, saying nothing.

"I began to think about my mother and father's death and the time when, after they died, I received news of my Uncle John T.'s death. I was startled then by how upset I was. I was startled now, as well, at how painful these memories still were. I thought I understood how Ann felt.

"Too tired to fix supper at home, I suggested we go out. Once seated at the restaurant, Ann mumbled something that I didn't catch. I said, 'What?'"

Ann interrupted Harold's story and said, "I said, 'Look here, stupid.' I glared at him and was almost shouting, as I pointed to a place on the menu that mentioned Livingston, Montana, where we had just vacationed. I was mad. I wasn't really mad at Harold. I was trying to get away from my grief, and I needed my anger to help me. It just happened that Harold was my target."

"I understood," Harold said, "because I have done the same thing to her many times. To defend myself, I said, 'I don't think you are mad at me. This anger covers up your tears for your uncle, right?'"

"My eyes filled with tears again," Ann said. "I just pulled the menu higher up to cover my face."

"My eyes filled up too, right along with hers. It was like you said, David. If we pay attention and try to understand, we find that we feel the same thing. When Ann grieved, I grieved with her. Somehow, because I knew what her anger meant, I felt our feelings somehow magically merge. Our tears were the same. This felt a lot better than being defensive and making your point."

The Neurology of Empathy/Compassion

We can easily speculate that there could be special parts of the brain that play a role in empathy, for example, the preoptic area of the hypothalamus. It is related to giving mating signals, nest building, and retrieving young who wander too far. In females, the medial preoptic area (MPOA) is more highly developed than in males (Fisher, 1964). The nucleus accumbens is particularly indicated as part of a tending circuit. This area contains an overlap of dopamine (DA) and oxytocin (OXY) receptors. In the limbic system, the thalamic circuitry is related to nursing and social play (MacLean, 1970). That system might offer promise for identifying specific brain circuits necessary for empathy.

OXY, a neurohormone, is related to compassion or empathy. Panksepp (1993) suggested it as "a prime candidate for mediating feelings of acceptance and social bonding" (p. 93).

Shelly Taylor (2001) was interested in whether there was a male/female difference in responses to stress. The male fight/flight response was well-documented. Taylor believed that females had a different response to our brain's red-alert mechanism in the amygdala. She found that difference in the brain's construction of the tending instinct. Under stress males tend to fight, females tend to nurture and protect. This is where we find a neurological basis for empathy and compassion.

Taylor (2001) found that while men tended to fight or flee in response to stress, women tended to seek social support. When Taylor (2001) studied male and female brains, she found oxytocin in both. But females had estrogen, which potentiates oxytocin, while testosterone in males does nothing to add to oxytocin's power. Vasopressin (VP) is the male analog to oxytocin. It is in both men and women, but it seems to be potentiated by testosterone. Vasopressin stimulates the male tending instinct to protect by fighting the threat.

In the prefrontal cortex two parts of the brain play a role in empathy. They are the orbital and medial frontal areas. These areas are active when one person is trying to figure out the intentions of another (Baron-Cohen, 2003).

Connected to this process of figuring out what's going on in the mind of another is superior temporal sulcus (STS) located in the temporal lobe. This area is also active when a person tries to look into the eyes of another and determine what's going on in that person's mind (Baron-Cohen, 2003). These areas are part of the large human brain that process feelings after they are registered in the feeling parts of the brain in the limbic system.

This makes the two different sexual responses to stress complementary. Females look for support when stressed. They reach out with a herding instinct to tend and care for, while males' instinct is to guard the herd. Both of these tendencies are nurturing, caretaking responses.

Studies of prairie voles document the importance of oxytocin in attachment bonds. The prairie vole, in contrast with the montane vole, mates for life. The prairie vole has a larger nucleus accumbens than the montane vole. The nucleus accumbens again is where the dopamine centers overlap the oxytocin centers. In the prairie vole, this places the bonding neurohormone smack in the center of the reward part of the brain. This then seems to strongly reward bonding (Carter, 1996).

The reptile brain does not produce oxytocin. Young reptiles do not require tending as mammalian young do. This is the evolutionary reason we humans tend to mate for life and have compassion for one another.

The Gift of Compassion

When compassion releases oxytocin, our immune system is activated. We become less tense, and we feel connected. Compassion that we feel for others reminds us of our social bonds. Compassion relieves us of our narcissism for a moment. It helps us see ourselves as part of, next to, rather than alone and disconnected. Compassion pushes us toward others and helps keep us involved with others. It can help give us the comforting feeling of being where we are supposed to be.

Freud is right to see compassion as part of the healthy development between parent and child. Darwin was also correct to see it as a species mechanism to help children survive. The nucleus accumbens serves to unite oxytocin and dopamine so that we get pleasure for tending and caring for others.

The Paradox of Oxytocin

Lactating mothers have higher amounts of oxytocin in their brains. Yes, it seems to calm stress and promote social connections. It elevates our immune system. It (along with dopamine) is the hormone most associated with love.

Most of the research on compassion/nurturing/tending speaks to its positive effects on the body (the enhancement of the immune system and the nurturing response to stress). The research holds the increase in oxytocin as the reason for these positive effects. But just as oxytocin is associated with love, it is also associated with the absence of love. This is the paradox of oxytocin. Taylor (2001) found high amounts of oxytocin in older women with nonsupportive, difficult husbands. She speculates that oxytocin triggers the drive toward social attachment. When the elderly woman feels crummy and needs support, oxytocin is released so that she will seek social affirmation. Oxytocin then is also associated with the need for affiliation.

Though there might or might not be one area of the brain that mediates empathy and compassion, clearly the brain is chemically equipped to tend, care for, anticipate, and understand another. Oxytocin is the chemical associated with compassion. We feel the feelings we see in the other. These feelings are contagious. This happens before we know it. This is how we tend to each other.

Empathy as a Brain Chemical

What does this mean about the flow of emotions from one to another? Yes, we can, by using our imaginations and being open to new feelings, find ways to push ourselves out of emotionally pathological places. But perhaps empathy, as a force, can do the same for us.

If we can get out of our self-absorption and focus on the feelings of those around us can naturally transform our brain neurohormones and turn on new emotional brain circuitry. Being willing to care about others and being emotionally a part of a community will, in and of itself, keep our emotional flow healthy. When we are depressed but our child successfully completes a piano recital and we look at her happy face, what happens inside our brains as we empathetically are filled with joy? Or consider another empathic moment: What happens to our brain chemistry and our brain circuitry when we have won, but see our opponent in tears?

This could be the reason that social networks are such positive influences on our health. This could be why sociable single women are so much healthier than socially isolated, divorced males; these women have a greater capacity for empathy and social connection (Antonucci, Lansford, & Sherman, 1998).

If feelings are naturally contagious, why do some of us share in communal feelings more easily than others? Baron-Cohen (2003) explained why there are sexual differences with the empathy reflex. People without regard to sex have different personality styles. Some of us merge our feelings with others easily, sometimes too easily. Those of us who merge easily often have trouble with social boundaries. Some of us don't know where we leave off and others begin. Possibly, we assume that everyone feels the same as we. Or, we get so caught up in the story of the other that we don't attend to our own. Still others of us are too bounded and well-defended. Those of us who are so well-defended don't care how others feel. We have built defenses that justify ignoring others. Disgust, anger, and pride play important roles in these defenses, as does respect, which is closely associated with fear.

My primary character flaw is how easily I merge with others. Boundaries have always seemed to me somewhat artificial and silly. When I was 5 years old, growing up in the summer heat of Arkansas, I wondered why people wore clothes. I didn't see the need for any defenses. My older brother, on the other hand, needed his space. He was careful with his possessions. He was neat and meticulous. He left my things alone and expected me to leave his alone. When Mother pleaded with him to understand his little brother, he would say, "I don't care how he feels." And I remember her pleading with me to leave his things alone. My reply was, "I would give him mine, if he wanted them." Only "mine" was never easy to find and not in very good shape when it was discovered.

The point is not that one personality style is better than the other. The point is that people differ in how available they are to another's feelings. We need to respect these differences—and I have tried to learn this. I feel fortunate in my work in that I have the ability to quickly and easily understand and love my clients. But this strength is also my therapeutic weakness. Too often, I want to help. Rather than believe my clients have the resources they need to solve their problems, I want to intrude in their lives. Luckily, my 15 years of therapy and supervision have kept me more or less on the correct side of the therapist/client boundary.

People naturally differ in their ability to establish boundaries and understand the feelings of others. In my case, it might be because I was the baby boy. In my brother's, it might have to do with his being a middle child. Whatever the reason, people differ on this dimension. I am more suggestible than my brother. Our personality styles bring us different good-and-bad consequences. I am a therapist because of my personality, and he is an excellent defense attorney because of his. He has friends, because he respects their autonomy, and I have friends, because I understand the other person's point of view. (Although my neighbors get mad at me when I don't remember to return their wheelbarrows.)

Empathy/compassion/tending is probably the personal strength and weakness of most therapists. How is empathy/compassion/tending defined? There are two versions of this psychological experience. One is the sympathy version. The other is empathy/compassion, with the addition of respect and boundaries. Sympathy uses the same emotional reflex of merging into the feelings of the other, but with a sense of superiority: "I pity him, poor thing;" "I feel sorry for her." These words have a condescending tone: "I'm not like them. I'm better than that;" "They hurt, because they are not as good as I am;" "That would never happen to me."

Healthy empathy/compassion/tending is not elitist. It is not "better than" or "different from." It is the same as: "Oh, my god, you must feel awful" (the implication being, "I would if I were you, and I am no better than you, that would hurt"); "I'll bet that was fun;" "I remember when my mother died. It felt as if the air went out of the world. Do you feel that way?" The boundary in healthy empathy/compassion comes from respect. Respect is the faith that the other person has the resources that she needs to solve her own problems. Her problem belongs to her not to us. She wants to be the one that solves her problems.

Compassion/empathy/sympathy gives us self-esteem. The sympathy version provides vertical self-esteem and helps us feel superior to someone else. The respect version does not make us feel better than someone else; it connects us to our friends and community. We feel a part of something more than just ourselves. We feel good about ourselves, because we are capable of understanding, caring, and connecting, not because we are superior. We see that our caring can matter to others and, that as we love and respect others, we are lovable.

Teaching Empathy/Compassion to Clients

Most therapists see couples as part of their practice. Communications skills are among the lessons therapists teach to both partners. When we do this, we are teaching empathy/compassion. Clients often are resistant to learning empathy, because they are afraid that if they really understand and care for another, they will be forced to put aside their own positions and give in to get along.

Of course, empathy/compassion has nothing to do with giving in. It has to do with understanding and validating feelings. We can understand how others feel and still maintain our feelings. We cannot lose our own experience or feelings. Once clients learn that they do not lose themselves when they listen, understand, and care for another, they easily learn how to use empathy/compassion in their discourse. The more they practice using empathy/compassion, the more competent they feel as social beings.

Empathy/compassion is indeed the master key of emotions. Becoming a master of understanding the other's point of view can help us past stubborn, angry adversaries. When we validate another person's reality and understand how that person feels, that individual often naturally reciprocates and listens to our sad story as their defenses against us diminish. This kind of compassionate sharing can help blend old, opposing realities into a new consensus.

Probably most therapists have versions of teaching empathy/compassion to clients. Carl Rogers and Robert Carkhuff teach empathy much more extensively that I do. I offer my version, because it is reduced to four easy-to-remember steps.

Love and empathy/compassion/tending are really the same. I use LOVE as my acronym to help clients remember the four steps essential to empathic/compassionate listening.

 Step 1: Listen. Pay attention to the person speaking. Listen for what that person feels. When you think you hear what he or she feels, mirror that emotion in your face, body language, and words. Repeat what you understand the speaker to say. Ask the person if you understand: "So, you feel afraid?"; "You seem happy."; "I can see that you're excited. Is that right?" You should always give the person you are listening to the position of authority on what he or she feels. As the listener, you should retain the position of wonder and curiosity about how the speaker feels. When you think

you know how the speaker feels, repeat this to the speaker so the speaker knows that you are trying to understand. When you begin to feel you are forgetting some of what that individual said, stop the narration and repeat what you understand so far. Then go on. The speaker will help you until you get it, because all of us yearn for understanding.

 Step 2: Offer understanding without blame. As you listen, do not shift the focus to your defense. Do not explain yourself. Really listening, caring, and empathizing means that you are not the focus of attention. Never blame or shame the speaker for feeling as he or she does. Of course, when you listen and reflect, you may sometimes use the words, "You are . . .". These words should never be followed by a name or label, for example, "You are a jerk." Be careful not to judge or talk about the individual's character in a blaming or shaming way. It is better to use the words, "you feel . . .", to introduce your response. Soon the speaker will see you are listening and you care, because you are not looking for a flaw in the speaker's reasoning or reasons for why this individual should feel differently. Instead, the speaker is feeling that you understand and that he or she has a right to feel the way they do. The speaker inevitably will relax and trust you as the listener. Listening without judgment or blame helps the speaker feel safe. Watching you eagerly trying to get it creates security.

 Step 3: Validate the speaker's feelings. This means saying something like, "I would feel that way too, if I were you." You can say that and still feel and see things differently, because you are not the speaker. But if you did see reality as this individual does (which you don't), you would feel the same. Of course, the speaker's experience causes him or her to feel this way. You would, too. When it is your turn to talk about how you feel, you can contrast your experience with the speaker's. But this is not the time for that. Now is the time to understand and validate the way his or her mind works. When you successfully validate that person's feelings, he or she naturally replies, "Yes, I have a right to feel what I feel, to be who I am. I'm not crazy. Thank God, and thank you for understanding."

 Step 4: Engage in change. Many times we can't fix what's wrong. We can't make the rain stop, but we can shift a bit to the left to make room for our clients under our umbrella. Harming yourself as you help another only brings resentment and guilt. But offering symbolic help and comfort lets you move in a different way. Maybe you can't right the wrong or fix the car, but you can bring flowers.

While they cope with personal tragedy, you can sweep their porch or fix a meal. You can write them a note. The speaker's pain can make a difference in how you behave. This is what love requires: real understanding and changing what you can, because you have listened and the other person matters to you.

Step 4, E, as I describe it here is meant for a client or for a part of a couple, not for a therapist. The therapist should avoid changing things in the client's world, but if a client feels hurt by something the therapist said or did, in addition to exploring the real source of the pain, the therapist might promise to try to avoid this behavior in the future.

Summary and Conclusion

It is important to emphasize some aspects of this ritual. As you use this exercise and become empathetically competent, notice that the speaker's defenses begin to drop when he or she feels understood and acknowledged. When you have your turn to talk with that person, he or she will be more open to understanding how you feel as well.

The most important thing you can do as you empathize with your partner is to help her believe that her feelings make sense. This is the essence of the third step, "V." We are all afraid that our feelings are irrational, and that we are crazy for feeling the way we do. It is a great gift when you say to your partner, "If I were you, I would feel just like you do. Your feelings make sense."

A final word of warning: In the first step, do not ask too much of yourself. You can listen only so long without being overloaded. When you begin to feel that you cannot remember all that your partner has said and cannot repeat all of it, interrupt and say, "I'm getting overloaded with information. Let me repeat to you what I understand you to have said so far." Then ask, "Is that what you are saying?" When your partner agrees that you have understood, ask your partner to continue.

My supervisor, Bob Stepbach, told me that the profession of therapist is one that could help make us better people, because part of our job is to focus on our own growth and development. I believe Bob was right for that reason and also because empathy cleanses the brain.

We can easily confuse empathy/compassion/tending with an emotion. Brain chemicals and brain structures support this instinct. The brain rewards us with pride and satisfaction when we use this response. It is essential to the survival of the species that we tend to each other and our young. But this tending involves understanding, caring for, and feeling with the object of our affection. The emotional content in our brain is the same as the person we are empathizing with. The difference is that the emotion is filtered through the part of our brain that engages our tending response. This is why, under stress, tending another lowers our stress, strengthens our immune system, and gives us a feeling of satisfaction and well-being. Compassion forms our emotional subtext to the feeling we experience with the person we are tending. It is as if we provide a constant beat to their music. We give them our consistent rhythm, as we take on their emotional melody. Both of us are comforted in the process.

Empathy/compassion is healing to relationships and communities. It brings with it warmth, tenderness, trust, and goodwill. But the greatest gift that empathy offers is to the brain of the person offering the empathy. It bathes the brain in a new set of emotional neurohormones. Therapists have the privilege of receiving this cleansing almost hourly. It is a gift to be able to channel love and compassion to another. This profession can make us better people because of the love-energy flowing through us. Aren't we therapists fortunate?

Getting back to Ann and Harold:

"You know David," Harold said, "Seeing you helped us some, but that goofy LOVE ritual you gave us to practice helped the most."

"Yes," Ann added. "We practiced and got better. I didn't believe that marriage had to do with skill or that there was any skill in listening as long as you both had ears. Now I'm not afraid to tell Harold how I feel. And he doesn't seem to be afraid of my feelings."

"I'm not," Harold responded, "But in practicing that ritual, I realized your feelings were yours to fix, that I couldn't change hers, but I could understand them. And when I did understand them, her feelings seemed to change. Listening seems so simple and it is, but it's not. When you do it right, it's as if you find a secret key. It opens her to understanding and caring about me. And it makes me feel better about myself. Empathy serves many masters."

CHAPTER 15

Emotions
The Symphony of Psychotherapy

Overview

In this book, I have described the raw material for building emotional harmony. It is like describing a musical composition through its use of melody and chord structure, showing how one complements the other and how they combine to form a harmonious whole.

I certainly have not written a symphony. I barely have even touched on an emotional chord. This theory building and its connection to music has miles to go before its potential is exhausted. The next step needs to be taken by a psychologist/musician or musician/psychologist who can methodically explore the parallels between music and emotion and help us see what music has to teach us about feelings.

In the first chapter I mentioned how much overlap there is between music and feelings. Why would any of us listen to music if we were not expecting or hoping to be emotionally touched or moved? Surely music moves through the same emotional neurostructures I have described.

For each emotion, I have suggested one harmonious path out of the monotony and overuse of that emotion or emotional knot. There are others, perhaps millions of combinations of emotions, which can lead to health and psychological balance. Music probably has more to teach us about these paths than does biochemistry.

There are emotional texts and subtexts that make up our emotional state. For example, the text (or point) may be sadness at the death of a parent and the subtext (or counterpoint) might be joy and desire that is part of receiving an inheritance (and perhaps and even deeper subtext of shame for feeling that way).

Most of the time, people present the pose or the text of a smiling face and respond to "How are you?" with "I am fine." This attitude is reflected in the Morey-Churchill song for Disney's *Snow White,* "Whistle While You Work." While happiness is the text, therapists are usually interested in understanding the subtext.

Most people who consult therapists have one chronic feeling that switches during the day between text and subtext. All these emotional elements have parallels in music.

I previously described empathy as the emotional master key. A repeated note in music is part of the melody, as well as the rhythm. Rhythm is the foundation of music. In song or in prose, a repeated refrain, as in Martin Luther King's landmark speech, "I have a dream," gives the piece a meaningful structure. In therapy, repeating a patient's words and reflecting his or her feelings connects the therapist to the client.

Empathy can always be used to connect one emotion to another. An empathetic therapist with a healthy therapeutic alliance can say almost anything to a client and the client will respectfully receive the input. This is because empathy has established an underlying rhythm or beat, and the therapist's next remark—his next note—fits inside the context of the empathetic rhythm and becomes a part of the joint or shared emotional melody that the therapeutic relationship has created.

I was in a men's group in the 1970s. One of the members of that group was a talented pianist, Andy Bernstein (who is now a talented psychologist). Andy could play melodies extemporaneously that seemed to pour out of his hands. His notes and chords reflected his moods beautifully. One of the things he could do with a piano was describe or diagnose people.

One night, for the six members of our group, Andy sat at the piano, played a melody, and asked which one of us this spontaneous musical interlude described. We correctly named each individual he painted with his music. Something Andy picked up in his music accurately reflected the emotional tone of each of us. For me, it was a forthright, clear, no-doubting, "I know, follow me" attitude in his music that unmistakably described my spirit. It amazed me that Andy could combine music and emotions to understand and describe people diagnostically, without using pejorative psychiatric labels.

Bryan Sutton is an internationally known, contemporary guitarist based in Nashville. One blustery, raw, rainy March evening I was fortunate enough to hear him in concert. He introduced one of his numbers by talking about the bad news in the paper. He wanted in his next piece to offer a spirit of goodness to counter the evil that filled the news and the air about us. He titled the song,

The Good Deed. Imagine the emotion the song evoked. It didn't evoke joy, and that makes sense, because joy would be too self-indulgent for goodness. Nor did it evoke desire for the same reason, nor anger, nor fear, nor surprise, nor disgust, nor sleep, nor shame. Listening to the piece, the obvious emotion associated with Bryan's version of goodness was sadness. As I think about this, it makes sense that values like goodness, badness, ambition, and caution each have an associated emotion and perhaps a counterpart in music.

Our bodies, posture, and clothes we wear operate like musical instruments. Each instrument has its range of notes, but a composer might choose one or another to express a particular emotion. Trumpets can proclaim the joy of triumph. Trombones, tubas, and tympani can express anger. Strings can reflect sadness.

Ten-year-old girls in summer shorts are very good at laughter and joy. Teenage boys dressed in leather sitting on motorcycles can portray anger easily. Young adult women are often cast in movies where they scream in fear. Often we look at people, their posture and clothes, and sense an emotion emerging from them. It really does not require extra-sensory perception to feel the emotional auras that surround people, just as it doesn't take a great deal of musical talent to look at a tuba and imagine what mood it can create.

The preceding notions about text and subtext; rhythm and empathy; diagnosis with music of the emotional spirit that emerges from each of us; the emotion of human values; the way our bodies, posture, and clothes communicate feelings in a similar way to musical instruments—these notions suggest that there is much more to be understood and many more contributions that can be made considering each emotion as a note in a multitude of human symphonies.

A trademark of noted jazz musician Thelonious Monk was to insert a discordant note and transform it to become part of the harmony of the music. As mentioned earlier, this was also a quality of Beethoven's Ninth Symphony. Beethoven moved back and forth among many musical and emotional themes, writing notes that one might think incompatible into beautiful music. He moved from discord to resolution. If we psychotherapists understood emotions and how to use them like these masterful musicians, it would be easy for us to help our patients transform their seemingly discordant notes into music. The point, of course, is that no note is discordant if we can find the right place for it in a sequence with other notes.

I write about the musical connections to emotions because this is part of what led me to see discrete emotions as useful therapeutic tools, but more importantly because music and art are as important to understanding the human experience as is biology. The future of psychotherapy theory is in uniting the elements of art, biology, and psychotherapy as we offer ways to help our clients move toward psychological well-being and self-mastery.

Theoretical Summary

The theory I present here is rooted in common sense. It is this simple: We are always feeling something. Most of the time we are in emotionally steady states, such as mild interest or contentment (a low-level version of joy). Daily, sometimes momentarily, our feelings shift from one to the other, depending on the circumstances we confront.

Each emotion has its own dynamic. That dynamic has strengths to offer us and can also contribute to our problems. Individual emotions are like the individual notes on a scale: do, re, me, fa, so, la, te, do. They can be combined harmoniously or discordantly. Individual emotions can be resources to psychotherapists and clients if they understand how emotions work.

We have nine basic emotions. They are: anger, fear, sadness, shame, interest, joy, surprise, fatigue, and disgust. Each of these emotions serves an adaptive purpose. We need to use all of them at varying levels of intensity from time to time.

Psychopathology occurs when we get stuck in one emotion or in an emotional knot or cycle. There are healthy paths that we all can use to help us out of the paralysis of being in stuck one emotion or tied up in an emotional knot. In this book, I have described some of these paths, using emotions to resolve the unhealthy emotional knots. These paths require common sense and creative imaginings. They are not for all clients, but they can be helpful to many.

Integrating Psychotherapy, Science, and Art

Perhaps science and psychotherapy have communicated so poorly because we have continued to perpetuate the mind/body dualism. In this text, I assert that discrete emotions are chemical reactions in certain parts of the brain. Further, I write that to understand emotions, we must understand how they function in humans—and evaluate their potential dysfunction in human behavior in the context of the brain's neurological circuitry and biochemistry.

Emotion Rituals is the only text that integrates the clinical application of emotion theory with its biological base and suggests a direction, using music as the future template for helping understand and transform feelings. I hope that what I have described here will become obvious and that therapists will encourage the development of other texts that teach the collaborative use of medications and emotional resolutions to treat emotional knots. Someday, therapists might be so well versed in neurobiology that they will listen to a client describe his or her symptoms and immediately think about neurocircuits and neurohormones, as well as healthy emotional paths that resolve emotional knots or traps and perhaps emotional music that can transform dysfunction into harmony.

Perhaps in the future, art, science, and practice will support each other in treating emotional problems. But currently practitioners like me avoid prescribing medications whenever possible. We seek resources within our patients that they can draw on to heal themselves, because we are suspicious of medications and the imposition of what seems to be an unnatural remedy.

Putting emotion theory into practice, as this book attempts, can build a collaborative interdisciplinary dialogue, using emotional experience as the unifying force. Such collaborative dialogue can help build mutual trust and respect for medicine and psychotherapy. Perhaps this will create a common language that all of us can use to serve those who suffer emotionally.

Perhaps also in the future, psychologists and other mental-health professionals will understand the physiology of the brain well enough to suggest medication in combination with behavioral homework. A day might come when psychiatrists will understand human emotional behavior well enough to suggest behavioral homework *instead* of medication. We should not establish "guild" boundaries that prevent mental- health professionals from healing their clients.

Contribution to the Field

In *Emotion Rituals*, I attempt to contribute to therapists' professionalism on two levels. The first is theoretical. This book gives therapists tools to conceptualize their practice in a new way. Using this theory, they can use their own experiences and emotions as keys to unlock the door to their clients' pain. They can see the imagination, thought, feeling, and biochemistry collaborating to create feelings and understand what they are seeing. With this theory, they know what to do to move beyond emotional knots. With this theory, they can help themselves and teach their patients to do the same.

Freud, Jung, Reich, and Rogers have suggested that denial and repression only increase our psychological pain and that we should let emotions flow, whatever they are and wherever they came from. Our culture of the twenty-first century, however, tells us that there are some people that we hope will discover better ways to express their feelings, for example, sexual offenders, batterers, bullies, and others who consider themselves entitled, better-than, and special.

Helping people who are frightened and sad connect with their predatory emotions of anger, desire, and joy works. And that is where psychotherapists have had the most success. But psychology has done a poor job of helping aggressive predators behave appropriately. This theory offers something for each emotional dysfunction. What it offers are resources that we all have and few of us know completely how to use. And these "resources" are each one of our emotions.

The second contribution of *Emotion Rituals* is practical. Each of the techniques offered at the close of the emotion chapters are basic, concrete tools. We can use them ourselves, and we can teach them to our clients.

Each morning, my mother picked up her meditation book and her Bible. She read them and prayed, hoping that somehow her spirit would start the day on the right path. When I was taught meditation, my teacher suggested that I use this tool twice daily. The techniques I offer here should be used as my mother used prayer or others use meditation. We should help our clients select the emotions with which they need help. They are the emotions that they most often use and the ones they avoid. They can begin using at least a daily ritual. They can practice feeling this once-neglected feeling—or resolving this too-often-used feeling—using the ritual that will help them become adept at moving beyond their characteristic emotional knot.

In a later text, I intend to demonstrate how to diagnose those emotions with which people need help, using archetypal examples and clinical stories to demonstrate how these techniques might be effective. For the time being, I present these rituals together with their theoretical underpinnings.

- For anger, the HEART ritual resolves anger with sadness and caps it off with compassion.
- For fear, the CALMS ritual teaches self-soothing through relaxing the body, preparing the mind for the trance, then visiting the trance through meditation.
- For sadness, the ALIVE ritual resolves sadness by adding playful anger to sadness to create determined action toward an object of interest/ desire.
- For interest and shame, the PRIDE ritual is useful. This technique requires resolving an inappropriate, self-destructive want with shame, then resolving shame with pride (a version of joy).
- For joy, the HELP ritual reveals the basic feelings that are being hidden by joy. This technique makes being vulnerable easier by engaging community and social network resources, teaching social networking, and allowing us to show ritual practitioners where and how they need help.
- For surprise, the SEEK ritual weakens the defense of confusion, surprise, and wonder and promotes clear, concrete thinking and committed action.
- For fatigue, the AWAKE ritual helps those paralyzed by the trance. It uses our social frame of reference. It encourages awareness of the present moment, facing and feeling our more painful emotions, and getting help from friends as we need it.
- For disgust, the LIMIT ritual helps build tolerance, using not-knowing as a resource to resolve disgust's implicit prejudice.

- For compassion/empathy/tending, the LOVE ritual teaches understanding and validation of the feelings of another. It helps people transcend their internal narcissism and gives them a vacation—from themselves.

Changing Emotions Is the Point

Many of us are concerned that research often fails to demonstrate the effectiveness of psychotherapy (Strupp 1993; Bickman 1996, 1998). This might be because researchers have never focused on emotions as an outcome variable. Wouldn't it be interesting to determine if psychotherapy changed how patients manage the flow of their emotions? Do they control their anger better? Do they manage fear? Can they self-soothe better? Do they use pride to resolve shame? Are they happy to be held accountable? Research focused specifically on the patient's skills at managing emotional flow likely would yield provocative results. (In addition to posing questions about emotions, it would be important to study how psychotherapy changes the patient's social ecology, using Roger Barker's [1968] Ecological Psychology measures. But this is a different subject.)

Another concern about which we therapists often commiserate is the language we use to talk about what we do. We need to make what we do relevant and understandable to our clients *and* to the general public. Our research too often appears to be proving the obvious over and over, for example, research supporting the theory that people repeat behaviors that reward them. Statistics and percentiles have become suspect.

Psychologists create obscure terms using the excuse that scientific language must be precise so that experiments can be replicated. Often these terms appear to support the "guild" of psychology rather than communicate information, much in the way Latin used in legal language once separated lawyers from the public. Psychologists need a language precise enough to address scientific concerns and, at the same time, speaks to the public. Scientists can be precise when they speak of sadness, anger, or fear. And everybody understands what they mean. Researchers, therapists, clients, and the public are expert at interpreting a smile. And we all know what tears say. This language can be precise, useful in research and clinical practice, and still be accessible to "the every person." Using emotion language, we can "give psychology away" as well (Miller, 1963).

A third concern shared by many therapists has to do with how labeling affects our clients. We need to use terms that create a professional shorthand way of communicating. We all require categories in order to think, yet must these categories be medical terms that pathologize human experience into illnesses? Nicholas Hobbs (1975), former president of the American

Psychological Association and author of psychology's first edition of ethical principles, and others have suggested that labels can be pejorative. The terms "moron," "retarded," and now "special" demonstrate how the culture perverts labels to injure people. Most would agree that a word that is as common as "special" is an improvement over "moron." Words like sadness, fear, shame, anger and words like posture and knots could be used to describe adaptive and maladaptive behavior patterns. Because these terms come from every-day speech, we are less likely to pervert them. Many therapists cringe when they hear someone say, "Oh she's a borderline." We know that is therapese for bad person—jerk or worse. Sad, afraid, entranced, confused are words that we all experience and understand. This language does not imply disease or illness, yet this language can be precise enough to be used to prescribe medication.

My primary fear about the ideas presented in this book is that they will be used as another cookie-cutter approach to treatment: "Oh, you are depressed. Here, take this manual and come back next week." A beginning therapist, afraid of relating to his or her clients in a meaningful way, could push a manual at a patient that explains the ALIVE technique or the CALMS ritual without grasping the pain their client is experiencing.

There is no substitute for listening as part of building a therapeutic relation-ship. Though I might have offered an explanation for why certain cognitive behavioral techniques work, they will never work if therapists don't know how to listen. We therapists must know how to give a patient our eyes, ears, and hearts. Therapists must know how to build a healthy alliance. They must know how to let clients know that we are not above them, rather we are with them. We and our clients are all working on the same thing: How to manage ourselves and grow. The practice of psychotherapy will always be an art.

Good therapy does not come from a formula. Though to some I appear to provide formulae here, those who blindly apply these ideas will fail. Re-search might even suggest success because clients in their self-report do not want to speak badly of their well-intentioned, though ineffective helper who tried but never really "got it." Good therapy is a process of following, staying behind, providing the empathetic rhythm to a healthy relationship, listen-ing, understanding, and helping by continuing to turn the frame around our client's experience until the client sees it and says, "That's it! You understand and so do I."

Sometimes this requires that we help clients out of an emotional knot or help them move beyond a chronic emotional posture—and sometimes not. No one-size-fits-all approach to therapy exists.

Once, I gave a longtime client a manual for the ALIVE technique. The next time she returned, she shoved the manual in my face, saying, "You will not reduce my experience to a book. I will not be patronized by someone who pretends to know something I don't. I liked it when you listened to me and seemed to care about how I felt. I will not have you become my teacher. I want to learn from myself with your help. I did not come here to learn that you know and I don't. If that's what happens here, we will both fail."

The rituals I present here obviously would not help that client.

Implications for Treatment

This theory has many implications for treatment. One is that people can find help without having to endure the degradation of a medical diagnosis. Treatment plans can be created; therapists can consult with supervisors without using pejorative labels. The focus can be on feelings and postures and ways to untie knots. This can produce healthier and more productive treatment conferences, treatment plans, and better patient involvement in their growth and development.

But we should remember that only some patients find information useful in their treatment, while other patients will be treated satisfactorily with medications. Therapists cannot simply tell patients what to do and how to feel. Empathy remains the therapist's central healing and relationship-building tool. Yes, for some patients, this information will help them become independent of the therapist quickly. But for others, effective therapy will still take longer, sometimes much longer.

The implications for the mental-health economy—should therapy move in this direction—are myriad. Insurance companies can ask that therapists teach these skills based on a central emotion theory in group settings, thus making therapy cheaper and more effective for those able to learn and work in such environments. Human-resource planners can buy insurance that does not require medical-model treatment. Individuals can choose among treatment options that include informational group therapy, couples therapy, and long-term individual therapy.

Employers can be assured cost-effective treatment that fits their employees' needs, rather than the six-sessions-and-out managed care currently offers. The managed-care mental-health bureaucracy can be dismantled, because with an organized cafeteria of options, individuals can be trusted to choose what is best for them.

The paths I plot as healthy paths out of maladaptive emotional knots are not the only healthy paths. In fact, I would guess that there are ways that each emotion can be a healthy next step. For example, I suggest that shame will only deepen the hole of sadness, but when the sadness is self-pity, shame can challenge us to surrender the victim role.

A prominent 80-year-old political figure came to see me some months after his wife of 45 years died. He was crying often, having trouble sleeping, and did not want to resort to medication. His doctor son told him that I had developed some interesting techniques, and he wondered what I might recommend. As you might imagine, I suggested that he might find anger an effective resource to protect him against his deep grief and place a scab on his open wound.

He refused to entertain this idea. He could not be mad at his deceased wife. Oh, he understood that this was a common reaction of a grieving person, but it wasn't his. And he wouldn't begin to betray his wife's memory by projecting anger at her now. I then suggested that he be angry at God. Well, he didn't believe in God. He left without getting help from me.

In an earlier part of the book, I said that joy cannot redeem sadness very often. While I still believe this to be true, it was not true in the example of the grieving widower. A few weeks later, I saw him in the grocery store. He was with a woman friend. She was 42 and attractive.

"We are living together," he told me with a broad smile on his face. "I am a very lucky man." He pulled me aside while she was looking for something in another aisle. "What does she see in me?! I don't know. But we get in bed together and hold each other. She says that's enough for her. At night, we read poetry to each other, or we read aloud from a good book. I've not quit my grieving for Jane. And I don't want to. But somehow, right beside my sadness, is a happiness that I never imagined."

Though I could not have predicted this for him (and he wasn't expecting to fall in love again either), joy did rescue him from being drowned in his sadness.

Emotions give us humans perhaps our first experience of a paradox. While philosophers might still debate about whether or not absolutes exist, there is one clear universal human absolute: humans experience emotions. And there is one subject on which each of us is the absolute authority. And that subject is how we feel. No other person can credibly be the expert on how we feel. We know about our own internal emotional experience better than anyone else.

The paradox is that while we are the absolute authority on our own emotions, our emotions continually change. They never stay exactly the same. So while we may know ourselves better than anyone else, we are constantly changing, never in the exact same emotional place for long.

In democracies, an essential public liberty is that we have a right to feel, think, and say whatever we want. The same cannot be said for behavior. Behavior can put us in jail or in some instances our behavior can be punishable by death. We must be careful with what we do. We are free to feel, to imagine, to dream of all sorts of possibilities, if we do not use our feelings to motivate inappropriate dangerous behavior. It is necessary to protect the social fabric and the public safety to hold us accountable for how we behave. It is just as necessary for the public good and our collective creative spirit that we all have the right to feel and imagine all of our possible thoughts and feelings. Feeling our feelings, at the same time controlling our behavior, are goals of creative and responsible living.

From all that has preceded this conclusion, it is easy to make the case that emotion is primary and intelligence is secondary to human growth and development. While this may be true, this does not mean that there are no limits to our use of emotions. Emotions can motivate changes in our behavior. Their primary function is to give or withdraw energy to support various behaviors.

Recently I was seeing a woman who had been married for some time and who had fallen in love with someone other than her husband. Her husband was a tolerant, patient, kind man. He waited as she explored the potential of this new relationship. She defined her therapeutic task as "following her heart." And she did. What she was not prepared for was how often her heart would change. She moved out of her marital home. Then she moved back in. Then she moved out. Then she moved in again. She was following her heart. Her ambivalent behavior continued until her husband's patience was exhausted. He finally filed for divorce, and her lover became disinterested.

The point of this example is that we should not take our feelings too seriously. If we wait, our feelings will change. We should not act on each emotional impulse. Rather we should become students of our emotions, watching them, seeing how they flow and change, acting on them of course, but only after evaluating what they are saying to and about us.

In the movie *Castaway,* Tom Hanks's character reflects on his experience of being lost on a deserted tropical island. He said that it was easy to despair, believing that he was forever lost, but that each wave brought in something new, some new bit of information or equipment. Though he could not predict what was coming next, he began to see that the next wave was likely to bring him something that his mind could use creatively.

Our emotions serve this purpose. They are always bringing something new, a new direction, a disappointment, a fear, a victory, a new note, and/or a new song. We are fascinating objects of our own inquiry. But to begin the study of the self, we must understand the music that our emotions make, the harmonies and disharmonies. That has been the purpose of this book: to teach us that each emotion has a place in our daily lives and a time and purpose exists for each one. The more we practice an exercise that expands our emotional range, the more likely we are to master our feelings.

Notes

1. McMillan, D.W., "Sense of Community," in *Journal of Community Psychology* 24(4) (1996): 315–325.
2. Dissmell is an emotion described as "turning up one's nose at fools." For Tomkins, this was different than disgust. This distinction is too esoteric for our purposes.
3. Cantero, J., M. Atienza, C. Gomez, and R. Salas, "Spectral structure and brain mapping of human alpha activities in different arousal states," in *Neuropsychobiology*, 39, (1999): 110–116.
4. A list of neurohormones includes epinephrine, norepinephrine, isoproternol, albuterol, bitolteroh, terbutaline, ritodrine, isoetharine, salmeterol, pirbuterol, and levalbuterol. A listof neurotransmitters, includes dopamine, serotonin, acetycholine, gamma-amino butyric acid (GABA), glutamate, endorphins, enkephalins, dynorphins, substance P, and vasoactive intestinal peptide.
5. Part of the loyalty oath to the Duluth model is that it assumes that battering is an all-male disease. New data from other countries indicate that women resort to domestic violence more often than men. Women hit more frequently during domestic disputes than men, but their blows do not do the physical damage of the blows from men.
6. Yvonne Agazarian considers her fork-in-the-road technique to be much more complex and involved than the version I offer here. For a more complete rendition of her ideas, see her 1997 book *Systems-Centered Therapy for Groups*.
7. Much of what I learned about cognitive loops I adapted from attending an Yvonne Agazarian workshop and watching this master therapist at work.
8. This exercise is not for the chronically angry person or for anyone who confuses fantasy with reality.
9. Most labels for this emotion don't include desire. I do because it clarifies the drive function of this affect.
10. Earlier we noted that many people see important distinctions between shame and guilt. For us here, they mean the same thing and have the same neurological correlates.
11. What I know about EMDR I learned from Janis Christenson and Tom Nielson's presentations at the Nashville Psychotherapy Institute's monthly Friday meetings.

References

Adams, D. B. (1979). Brain mechanisms for offense, defense, and submission. *The Behavioral and Brain Sciences, 2,* 210–43.

Agazarian, Y. M. (1995). *The visible and invisible group: Two perspectives on group psychotherapy and group process.* London: Kamac Books.

Agazarian, Y. M. (1997). *Systems-centered therapy for groups.* New York: Guilford Press.

Allan, R., & Scheidt, S. (1996). *Heart & mind: The practice of cardiac psychology.* Washington, DC: American Psychological Association.

Antonijevic, I., Murck, H., Frieboes, R. F., Barthelmes, J., & Steiger, A. (2000). Sexually dimorphic effects of GHRH on sleep-endocrine activity in patients with depression and normal controls: Part I: The sleep EEG. *Sleep Research Online, 3*(1), 5–13.

Antonucci, T., Lansford, J., & Sherman, A. (1998). Satisfaction with social networks: An examination of socioemotional selectivity theory across cohorts. *Psychology and Aging, 13*(4), 544–552.

Aristotle. (1941). *The basic works of Aristotle* (R. McKeon, Ed.). New York: Random House.

Atkinson, B. 1999. The emotional imperative. *Family Therapy Networker, 23*(4), 22–33.

Austin, J. H. (1998). *Zen and the brain: Toward an understanding of meditation and consciousness.* Cambridge, MA: MIT Press.

Bandura, A. (1973). *Aggression: A social learning analysis.* Englewood Cliffs, NJ: Prentice Hall.

Barker, R. G. (1968). *Ecological psychology: Concepts and methods for studying the environment of human behavior.* Stanford University Press.

Baron-Cohen, S. (2003). *The essential difference: The truth about the male and female brain.* New York: Basic Books.

Batson, D., Batson, J., Slingsby, J., Harrell, K., Peekna, H., & Todd, R. M. (1991). Empathetic joy and the empathy-altruism hypothesis. *Journal of Personality and Social Psychology, 61,* 413–423.

Baumesiter, R. F., Smart, L., & Boden, J. M. (1996). Relation of threatened egotism to violence and aggression: The dark side of high self-esteem. *Psychological Review, 103,* 5–33.

Benelli, A., Poggioli, R., Luppi, P., Ruini, L., Bertolini, A., & Arletti, R. (1994). Oxytocin enhances, and oxytocin antagonism decreases, sexual receptivity in intact female rats. *Neuropeptides, 27,* 245–250.

Bennett, W. (1998). *Death of outrage: Bill Clinton and the assault on American ideals.* New York: Simon & Schuster.

Benson, H. (1975). *The relaxation response.* New York: Morrow.

Benson, H., Alexander, S., & Feldman, C. L. (1975). Decreased premature ventricular contractions through use of relaxation response in patients with stable ischaemic heart disease. *Lancet, 2,* 380–382.

Bernstein, D. A., & Borkovec, T. D. (1973). *Progressive relaxation training.* Champaign, IL: Research Press.

Bickman, L. (1996). A continuum of care: More is not always better. *American Psychologist,* Vol. 51(7), 689–701.

Boiten, F. (1996). Autonomic response patterns during voluntary facial action. *Psychophysiology,* 33, 123–131.

Bradley, M., Lang, P., & Cuthbert, B. (1993). Emotion, novelty, and the startle reflex: Habituation in humans. *Behavioral Neuroscience,* 107(6), 970–980.

Bradwejn, J. (1993). Neurobiological investigations into the role of cholecystokinin in panic disorder. *Journal of Psychiatry & Neuroscience,* 18, 178–188.

Bremer, F. (1935). Cerveau "isole" et physiologie du sommeil [The "isolated" brain and the physiology of sleep]. *Comptes Rendus des Searres,* 118, 1235–1241.

Buck, R. (1988). *Human motivation and emotion* (2nd ed.). New York: Wiley.

Buck, R. (1999). The biological affects: A typology. *Psychological Review,* 106(2), 301–336.

Buck, R., Lasaw, J., Murphy, M., & Costanzo, P. (1992). Social facilitation and inhibition of emotional expression and communication. *Journal of Personality and Social Psychology,* 6(6), 301–336.

Byl, N. N., Merzenich, M. M., & Jenkins, W. M. (1996). A primate genesis model of focal dystonia and repetitive strain injury. I. Learning-induced dedifferentiation of the representation of the hand in the primary somatosensory cortex in adult monkeys. *Neurology,* 47, 508–520.

Byl, N. N., Nagarajan, S., & McKenzie, A. (2000). Effect of sensorimotor training on structure and function in three patients with focal hand dystonia. *Society for Neuroscience Abstracts.*

Cacioppo, J. T. (2000). *The Handbook of Psychophysiology.* Cambridge University Press.

Cacioppo, J. T., Tassinary, L. G., & Fridlund, A. (1990). The skeletomotor system. In J. T. Cacioppo & L. G. Tassinary (Eds.), *Principles of psychophysiology: Physical, social, and inferential elements* (pp. 325–384). New York: Cambridge University Press.

Cahill, L. (1996). Neurobiology of memory for emotional events: Converging evidence from infra-human and human studies. *Cold Spring Harbor Symposia on Quantitative Biology,* 61, 259–264.

Caldwell, J. D., Johns, J. M., Faggin, B. M., Senger, M. A., & Pederson, C. A. (1994). Infusion of an oxytocin antagonist into the medial peoptic area prior to progesterone prohibits sexual receptivity and increases rejection in female rats. *Hormone Behavior,* 28, 288–302.

Candia, V., Elbert, T., Altenmuller, E., et al (1999). Constraint-induced movement therapy for focal hand dystonia in musicians. *Lancet, 353,* 42.

Cannon, W. B. (1927). The James-Lange theory of emotion: A critical examination and an alternative theory. *American Journal of Psychology,* 39, 106–124.

Cantero, J., Atienza, M., Gomez, C., & Salas, R. (1999). Spectral structure and brain mapping of human alpha activities in different arousal states. *Neuropsychobiology,* 39, 110–116.

Carkhuff, R. (1969). *Helping human relations: A primer for lay and professional helpers* (Vol. 2). New York: Holt, Rinehart & Winston.

Carter, C. S. (1996). *Peptides, steroids, and pairbonding.* Paper presented at the New York Academy of Sciences Conference on the Integrative Neurobiology of Affiliation, Georgetown University, Washington, DC.

Chevalier-Skolnikoff, S. (1973). Facial expression of emotion in nonhuman primates. In P. Ekman (Ed.), *Darwin and facial expression: A century of research in review* (pp. 11–90). New York: Academic Press.

Chwalisz, K., Diener, E., & Gallagher, D. (1988). Autonomic arousal feedback and emotional experience: Evidence from the spinal cord injured. *Journal of Personality and Social Psychology,* 54, 820–828.

Cicchetti, D., & Toth, S. L. (1998). Perspectives on research and practice in developmental psychopathology. In W. Damon (Series Ed.), I. Sigel, & K. A. Renninger (Vol. Eds.), *Handbook of child psychology: Vol. 4. Child psychology in practice* (5th ed., pp. 479–583). NewYork: Wiley.

D'Aquili, E. G., & Newberg, A. B. (1999). *The mystical mind: probing the biology of religious experience (theology and sciences).* Minneapolis, MN: Augsburg Fortress Press.

Damasio, A. R. (1994). *Descartes' error: Emotion, reason, and the human brain.* New York: Putnam.

Damasio, A. R. (2000). *The feeling of what happens: Body and emotion in the making of consciousness.* New York: Harcourt Brace & Company.

Darwin, C. R. (1965). *The expression of the emotions in man and animals.* Chicago: University of Chicago Press. (Original work published in 1872.)

Davidson, R. J. (1992). Emotion and affective style: Hemispheric substrates. *Psychological Science, 3,* 39–43.

Davidson, R. J. (1993). The neuropsychology of emotion and affective style. In M. Lewis & J. M. Haviland (Eds.), *Handbook of emotions* (pp. 143–154). New York: Guilford Press.

Davidson, R., Ekman, P., Saron, C., & Senulis, J. (1990). Approach, withdrawal, and cerebral asymmetry: Emotional expression and brain physiology. *Journal of Personality & Social Psychology, 58*(2), 330–341.

Dawson, M., Hazlett, E., Filion, D., & Nuechterlein, K. (1993). Attention and schizophrenia: Modulation of the startle reflex. *Journal of Abnormal Psychology, 102*(4), 633–641.

De Waal, F., & Aureli, F. (1997). Conflict resolution and distress alleviation in monkeys and apes. In C. S. Carter, I. I. Lederhendler, & B. Kirkpatrick (Eds.), *Annals of the New York Academy of Sciences: Vol. 807. The integrative neurobiology of affiliation* (pp. 317–328). New York: New York Academy of Sciences.

Demaree, H. A., & Harrison, D. W. (1997). A neuropsychological model relating self-awareness to hostility. *Neuropsychology Review, 7,* 171–185.

Derryberry, D., & Tucker, D. (1992). Neural mechanisms of emotion. *Journal of Consulting and Clinical Psychology, 60*(3), 329–338.

Descartes, R. (1989). *On the passions of the soul* (S. Voss, Trans.). Indianapolis, IN: Hackett. (Original work published 1649.)

Dollard, J., & Miller, N. E. (1950). *Personality and psychotherapy.* New York: McGraw-Hill.

Douglas, M. (1966). *Purity and danger.* London: Routledge & Kegan Paul.

Easterling, D., & Leventhal, H. (1989). Contributions of concrete cognition to emotion: Neutral symptoms as elicitors of worry about cancer. *Journal of Applied Psychology, 74*(5), 787–796.

Edelman, R. J. (1987). *The psychology of embarrassment.* Chichester, UK: Wiley.

Ekman, P. (1977). Biological and cultural contributions to the body and facial movement. In J. Blacking (Ed.), *The anthropology of the body* (pp. 34–84). London: Academic Press.

Ekman, P. (1994). Strong evidence for universals in facial expressions: A reply to Russell's mistaken critique. *Psychological Bulletin, 115,* 268–287.

Ekman, P., Levenson, R. W., & Friesen, W. V. (1983). Autonomic nervous system activity distinguishes among emotions. *Science, 221,* 1208–1210.

Ellsworth, P. C. (1994). William James and emotion: Is a century of fame worth a century of misunderstanding? *Psychological Review, 101,* 222–229.

Erickson, M., Rossi, E., & Rossi, S. (1976). *Hypnotic realities.* New York: Irvington.

Fanselow, M. S. (1994). Neural organization of the defense behavior system responsible for fear. *Psychonomic Bulletin Reviews, 1,* 429–438.

Ferguson, T., Stegge, H., Miller, E., & Olsen, M. (1999). Guilt, shame and symptoms in children. *Developmental Psychology, 35*(2), 347–357.

Fetterman, G. (1996). Dimensions of stimulus complexity. *Journal of Experimental Psychology: Animal Behavior Processes, 22*(1), 3–18.

Fisher, A. E. (1964). Chemical stimulation of the brain. *Scientific American, 210,* 60–69.

Fox, N. (1991). If it's not the left, it's the right: Electroencephalograph asymmetry and the development of emotions. *American Psychologist, 46*(8), 863–872.

Fox, R. E. (2003, August). *Toward creating a real profession of psychology.* Paper presented at the Annual Meeting of the American Psychological Association, Toronto, Ontario, Canada.

Frankland, P., & Yoemans, J. (1995). Fear-potentiated startle and electrically evolved startle mediated by synapses in rostrolateral midbrain. *Behavioral Neuroscience, 109*(4), 669–680.

Fredrickson, B. (2001). Broaden and Build theory. *American Psychologist, 56*(3), 218–226.

Freud, S. (1935). *The unconscious* (C. M. Baines, Trans.). In essays in metapsychology. London: Liveright. (Original work published 1915.)

Freud, S. (1936). *The ego and mechanism of defense.* London: Hogarth Press.

Freud, S. & Breuer, J. (1949). On the psychical mechanism of hysterical phenomena: A preliminary communication. In J. Strachey (Ed.), *Sandard edition* (Vol. 2, 1–13). London: Hogarth Press (Original work published 1893.)

Frijda, N. H.(1986). *The emotions.* Cambridge: Cambridge University Press.

Gendlin, E. T. (1996). *Focusing-oriented psychotherapy: A manual of the experiential method.* New York: Guilford Press.

Geppert, U. (1986). *A coding system for analyzing behavioral expressions of self-evaluative emotions.* Munich: Max-Planck-Institute for Psychological Research.

Gilbert, D., & Wilson, T. D. (2000). Miswanting: Some problems in the forecasting of future affective states. In J. Forgas (Ed.), *Thinking and feeling: The role of affect in social cognition.* Cambridge: Cambridge University Press.

Glaus, K., & Schwartzman, J. (2000). Depression and coronary heart disease in women: Implications for clinical practice and research. *Professional Psychology: Research and Practice, 31*(1), 48–57.

Gottman, J. M., Katz, L. F., & Hooven, C. (1997). *Meta-emotion: How families communicate emotionally.* Mahwah, NJ: Erlbaum.

Graffin, N., Ray, W., & Lundy, R. (1995). EEG concomitants of hypnosis and hypnotic susceptibility. *Journal of Abnormal Psychology, 104*(1), 123–131.

Gray, J. A. (1977). Drug effects on fear and frustration: Possible limbis site of action of minor tranquilizers. In L. L. Iverson, S. D. Iverson & S. H. Snyder (Eds.), *Handbook of psychopharmacology: Vol 8. Drugs, neurotransmitters, and behavior* (pp. 171–197). New York: Plenum.

Greenberg, L. S. (2001). *Emotion-focused therapy.* American Psychological Association: Washington, DC.

Greenberg, L. S. (2002). *Emotion-focused therapy.* American Psychological Association: Washington, DC. (Second Printing).

Greenberg, L. S., & Paivio, S. C. (1997). *Working with emotions in psychotherapy.* New York: Guilford Press.

Greenberg, L. S., & Safran, J. D. (1987). *Emotion in psychotherapy.* New York: Guilford Press.

Greenberg, L. S., & Safran, J. D. (1991). *Emotion, psychotherapy, and change.* New York: Guilford Press.

Haidt, J. (2000). The positive emotions of elevation. *Prevention and Treatment, 3,* Retrieved January 20, 2001, from http://www.journals.aga.org/prevention/volume3/ pre0030003c.html.

Harrell, A. (1991). *Evaluation of court-ordered treatment for domestic violence offenders: Final report.* (State Justice Institute Grant # 90-12L-E-089.)

Heller, W. (1993). Neuropsychological mechanism of individual differences in emotion, personality and arousal. *Neuropsychology, 7*(4), 476–489.

Hess, W.R. (1957). *Functional organization of the diencephalon.* New York: Grune & Stratton.

Hobbs, N. (1975). *The Futures of Children.* San Francisco: Jossey-Bass.

Hume, D. (1739). *Treatise on human nature.* London: John Noon.

Insel, T. R. (1992). Oxytocin: A neuropeptide for affiliation—evidence from behavioral, autoradiographic and comparative studies. *Psychoneuroendocrinology, 17,* 13–35.

Izard, C. E. (1971). *The face of emotion.* New York: Appleton-Century-Crofts.

Izard, C. E. (1972). *Patterns of emotion: a new analysis of anxiety and depression.* New York: Academic Press.

Izard, C.E. (1991). *The psychology of emotions.* New York: Plenum.

Izard, C. & Ackerman, B. (1999). Motivational, organizational, and regulatory functions of discrete emotions. *Handbook of Emotions* (2nd ed., pp. 253–264). New York: Guilford Press.

James, W. (1884). What is an emotion? *Mind*, 9, 188–205.

Janov, A. (1970). *The primal scream*. New York: Dell.

Johnson, S. (2004). *Mind wide open: Your brain and the neuroscience of everyday life*. New York: Scribner.

Joiner, T. (1994). Contagious depression: Existence, specificity to depressed symptoms and the role of reassurance seeking. *Journal of Personality & Social Psychology*, 67(2), 287–296.

Jung, C. G. (1946). Psychological types. In H. Read, M. Fordham, & G. Adler (Eds.), *The collected works of C. G. Jung* (Vol. 6). New York: Pantheon Books.

Jung, C. G. (1953). Two essays on analytical psychology. In H. Read, M. Fordham, & G. Adler (Eds.), *The collected works of C. G. Jung* (Vol. 7). New York: Pantheon Books

Kandel, E. (2001). The molecular biology of memory storage: A dialogue between genes and synapses. *Science*, 294, 1030–1038.

Kant, I. (1953a). *Critique on judgement* (J. H. Bernard, Trans.). New York: Harner. (Original work published 1938.)

Kant, I. (1953b). *Critique of pure reason* (N. K. Smith, Trans.). London: MacMillan.

Keltner, D., & Ekman, P. (1996). Affective intensity and emotional responses. *Cognition and Emotion*, 10(3), 323–328.

Koolhaas, J., van den Brink, T., Roozendaal, B., & Boorsma, F. (1990). Medial amygdala and aggressive behavior: Interaction between testosterone and vasopressin. *Aggressive Behavior*, 16, 223–229.

Kramer, P. D. (1993). *Listening to Prozac*. New York: Viking.

Kübler-Ross, E. (1969). *On death and dying*. New York: Macmillan.

Kugler, K., & Jones, W. (1992). On conceptualizing and assessing guilt. *Journal of Personality and Social Psychology*, 62(2), 318–327.

Laing, R. D., (1972). *Knots*. Random House Trade Paperbacks.

Lang, P., Bradley, M., & Cuthbert, B. (1990). Emotion, attention, and the startle reflex. *Psychological Review*, 97, 377–395.

Lange, C. G. (1885). *Om sindsbevaegelser: Et psyko-fysiologisk studie*. Kjbenhavn: Jacob Lunds. Reprinted in *The emotions*. C. G. James and W. James (Eds.), I. A. Haupt (Trans.) Baltimore, Williams & Wilkins Company. (Original work published 1922.)

Langer, L. (1958). *The symbolism of reason, rite and art*. New York: Mentor Books.

LeGros, J., Clark, W., Beattie, J., Riddoch, G., & Dott, N. (1938). *The hypothalamus*. Edinburgh, Scotland: Oliver & Boyd.

LeDoux, J. E. (1996). *The emotional brain*. New York: Simon & Schuster.

Levant, R. F. (2003). The Empirically-Validated Treatments Movement: A Practitioner Perspective. *Psychotherapy Bulletin, Vol. 38*(3), 36–39.

Levenson, R. W. (1992). Autonomic nervous system differences among emotions. *Psychological Science*, 3, 23–27.

Levenson, R., Ekman, P., & Friesen, W. (1990). Voluntary facial action generates emotion-specific autonomic nervous system activity. *Psychophysiology*, 27, 363–384.

Levenson, R., Carstensen, L., Friesen, W., & Ekman, P. (1991). Emotion, physiology, and expression in old age. *Psychology and Aging*, 6, 28–35.

Levenson, R., Ekman, P., Heider, K., & Friesen, W. (1992). Emotion and autonomic nervous system activity in the Minangkabau of West Sumatra. *Journal of Personality and Social Psychology*, 62, 972–988.

Lewis, H. B. (1971). *Shame and guilt in neurosis*. New York: International Universities Press.

Lewis, M. (1995). *Shame: The exposed self*. New York: The Free Press.

Lindsley, D. B. (1951). Emotion. In S. S. Stevens (Ed.), *Handbook of experimental psychology* (pp. 473–516). New York: Wiley.

Lindsley, D. B. (1957). Psychophysiology and motivation. In M. R. Jones (Ed.), *Nebraska Symposium on Motivation, 5* (pp. 44–105). Lincoln: University of Nebraska Press.

Loeb, E. (1991). *Joy*. White Plains, NY: Peter Pauper Press, Inc.

248 • References

Lorenz, K. (1950). Part and parcel in animal and human societies. In K. Lorenz (Ed.), *Studies in animal and human behavior* (Vol. 2, pp. 115–195). London: Methuen.
Loumaye, E., Thorner, J., & Cutt, K. J. (1982). Yeast mating pheromone activates mammalian gonado-tropins: Evolutionary conservation of a reproductive hormone? *Science, 218*, 1323–1325.
Lowenstein, G., & Schkade,D. (1999). "Wouldn't it be Nice? Predicting Future Feelings." In Kahne-man, D., Diener, E., & Schwartz, N. (Eds.), *Well-being: The foundations of hedonic psychology.* New York: Russell Sage.
Luu, P., Collins, P., & Tucker, D. (2000). Mood, personality, and self-monitoring negative affect and emotionality in relation to frontal lobe mechanisms of error monitoring. *Journal of Experimental Psychology, 129*(1), 43–60.
Maas, J. W. (1975). Biogenic amines and depression: Biochemical and pharmacological separation of two subtypes of depression. *Archives of General Psychiatry, 32*, 1357–1361.
MacLean, P. D. (1970). The limbic brain in relation to psychoses. In P. H. Black & M. B. Arnold (Eds.), *Physiological correlates of emotion* (pp. 659–678). New York: Academic Press.
MacLean, P. D. (1973). *A triune concept of the brain and behaviour.* Toronto: University of Toronto Press.
MacLean, P. D. (1993). Cerebral evolution of emotion. In M. Lewis & J. Haviland (Eds.), *Handbook of emotions* (pp. 67–83). New York: Guilford Press.
Maguire, E. A., Gadian, D. G., Johnsrude, I. S., Good, C. D., Ashburner, J., Frackowiak, R. S. J., & Frith, C. D. (2000). Navigation-related structural change in the hippocampi of taxi drivers. *PNAS, 97*, 4398–4403.
Mahrer, A. H. (1978). *Experiencing: A humanistic theory of psychology and psychiatry.* New York: Brunner/Mazel
Maier, S., Grahn, R., Kalman, B., Sutton, L., Wiertelak, E., & Watkins, L. (1993). The role of the amygdala and dorsal raphe nucleus in mediating the behavioral consequences of inescapable shock. *Behavioral Neuroscience, 107*(2), 377–388.
McCullough, M. E., Kilpatrick, S. D., Emmons, R. A. & Larson, D. B. (2001). Is gratitude a moral affect? *Psychological Bulletin, 127*, 249–266.
McEwen B. S., & Sapolsky R. M. (1995). Stress and cognitive function. *Current Opinion in Neuro-biology, 5*, 205–216.
McGaugh, J., Mesches, M., Cahill, L., Parent, M., Coleman-Mesches, K., & Salinas, J. (1995). Involve-ment of the amygdala in the regulation of memory storage. In McGaugh, F. Bermudez-Rattoni & R. A. Prado-Alcala (Eds.), *Plasticity in the central nervous system* (pp. 18–39). Hillsdale, NJ: Erlbaum.
McWilliams, N. (1994). *Psychoanalytic diagnosis.* New York: Guilford Press.
Merzenich, M. (2000). Seeing in the sound zone. *Nature, 404*, 820–821.
Miller, G. A. (1963). *Giving Psychology Away.* Eastern Psychological Association: Presidential Ad-dress 1969.
Miller, W. I. (1997). *The anatomy of disgust.* Cambridge, MA: Harvard University Press.
Miller, B. D., & Wood, B. L. (1997). Influence of specific emotional states on autonomic reactivity and pulmonary function in asthmatic children. *Journal of the American Academy of Child and Adolescent Psychiatry, 36*, 669–677.
Miller, A., Miller, R., Obermeyer W., Behan, M., &, Benca, R. (1999). The pretectum mediates rapid eye movement sleep regulation by light. *Behavioral Neuroscience, 113*(4), 755–765.
Mischel, W., & Peake, P. (1990). Predicting adolescent cognitive and self-regulatory competencies from pre-school delay of gratification. *Developmental Psychology, 26*(6), 978–986.
Moore, F. L. (1987). Behavioral actions of neurohypophysial peptides. In D. Crews (Ed.), *Psycho-biology of reproductive behavior: An evolutionary perspective* (pp. 61–87). Englewood Cliffs, NJ: Prentice Hall.
Morgan, M., & LeDoux, J. (1995). Differential contribution of dorsal and ventral medial prefrontal cortex to the acquisition and extinction of conditioned fear. *Behavioral Neuroscience, 109*, 681–688.

Morgan, M., Romanski, L., & LeDoux, J. (1993). Extinction of emotional learning: Contribution of medial prefrontal cortex. *Neuroscience Letters, 163,* 109–113.

Napier, T. C., Kalivas, P. W., & Hanin, I. (Eds.) (1991). *The basal forebrain: Anatomy to function.* New York: Plenum Press.

Nasar, S. (1998). *Beautiful mind.* New York: Simon & Schuster.

Nathanson, D. (1990). Project for the study of emotion. In R. A. Glick & S. Bone (Eds.), *Pleasure beyond the pleasure principle: The role of affect in motivation, development, and adaptation* (pp. 81–110). New Haven, CT: Yale University Press.

Nathanson, D. L. (1992). *Shame and pride: Affect, sex, and the birth of the self.* New York: W. W. Norton.

National Advisory Mental Health Council (1995). Basic behavioral science research for mental health: A national investment in emotion and motivation. *American Psychologist, 50*(10), 838–845.

Newbrough, J. R. (1995). Toward community: A third position. *American Journal of Community Psychology, 23,* 9–31.

Newman, S. W., Parfitt, D., & Kollack-Walker, S. (1997). Mating-induced c-fos expression patterns complement and supplement observations after lesions in the male syrian hamster brain. In C. S. Carter, I. I. Lederhendler, & B. Kirkpatrick (Eds.), *Annals of the New York Academy of Sciences: Vol. 807. The integrative neurobiology of affiliation* (pp. 239–259). New York: New York Academy of Sciences.

Nietzsche, F. (1967). *On the genealogy of morals* (W. Kaufmann, Trans.). New York: Random House. (Original work published 1887.)

Norcross, J. C. (2001). Purposes, processes, and products of the Task Force on Empirically Supported Theory Relationships. *Psychotherapy: Theory/Research/Practice/Training, 38,* 345–356.

Novaco, R. W. (1997). Remediating anger and aggression with violent offenders. *Legal and Criminal Psychology, 2,* 77–88.

Numan, M. (1996). *The neuroanatomical circuitry for mammalian behavior.* Paper presented at the New York Academy of Sciences Conference on the Integrative Neurobiology of Affiliation, Georgetown University, Washington, DC.

Olds, J. (1977). *Drives and reinforcement.* New York: Raven Press.

Olds, M., & Olds, J. (1963). Approach-avoidance analysis of the rat diencephalon. *Journal of Comparative Neurology, 120,* 259–295.

Olson, J. (2001). *Clinical pharmacology made ridiculously simple.* Miami, FL: MedMaster.

Orr, S., Lasko, N., Arieh, Y., & Pitman, R. (1995). Physiologic responses to load tones in Vietnam veterans with posttraumatic stress disorder. *Journal of Abnormal Psychology, 104*(1), 75–82.

Paivio, S., & Greenberg, L. S. (2001). Introduction to special issue on treating emotion regulation problems in psychotherapy. *In-Session, 57,* 153–156.

Panksepp, J. (1981). Hypothalamic integration of behavior. In P. Morgane & Panksepp (Eds.), *Handbook of the hypothalamus* (pp. 289–487). New York: Marcel Bekker.

Panksepp, J. (1982). Toward a general psychobiological theory of emotions. *The Behavioral and Brain Sciences, 5,* 407–467.

Panksepp, J. (1986). The neurochemistry of behavior. *Annual Review of Psychology, 37,* 77–107.

Panksepp, J. (1991). Affective neuroscience: A conceptual framework for the neurobiological study of emotions. In K. Strongman (Ed.), *International review of emotion research* (Vol. 1, pp. 59–99). Chichester, UK: Wiley.

Panksepp, J. (1992). A critical role for "affective neuroscience" in resolving what is basic about basic emotions. *Psychological Review, 99,* 554–560.

Panksepp, J. (1993). Neurochemical control of moods and emotions: Amino acids to neuropeptides. In M. Lewis & J. Haviland (Eds.), *Handbook of emotions* (pp. 57–107). New York: Guilford Press.

Panksepp, J. (1996). Affective neuroscience: A paradigm to study the animate circuits for human emotions. In R. Kavanaugh, B. Zimmerberg, & S. Fein (Eds.), *Emotion: Interdisciplinary perspectives* (pp. 29–60). Mahwah, NJ: Erlbaum.

Panksepp, J. (1998). *Affective neuroscience: The foundations of human and animal emotions.* New York: Oxford University Press.

Panksepp, J., Nelson, E., & Bekkedal, M. (1997). Brain systems for the mediation of social separation-distress and social reward: Evolutionary antecedents and neuropeptide intermediaries. In C. S. Carter, I. I. Lederhendler, & B. Kirkpatrick (Eds.), *Annals of the New York Academy of Sciences: Vol. 807. The integrative neurobiology of affiliation* (pp. 78–100). New YorK: New York Academy of Sciences.

Panksepp, J., Siviy, S., & Normansell, L. (1984). The psychobiology of play: Theoretical and methodological perspectives. *Neuroscience and Behavioral Reviews, 8,* 465–492.

Panksepp, J., Sacks, D., Crepeau, L., & Abbott, B. (1991). The psycho- and neuro-biology of fear systems in the brain. In M. R. Denny (Ed.), *Aversive events and behavior* (pp. 7–59). Hillsdale, NJ: Erlbaum.

Papez, J. W. (1937). A proposed mechanism of emotion. *Archives of Neurology and Psychiatry, 38,* 725–743.

Perls, F. S. (1947). *Ego, Hunger and Aggression.* London: George Allen & Unwin.

Persinger, M. A. (2002). Experimental simulation of the god experience: Implications for religious beliefs and the future of the human species. In R. Joseph (Ed.). *Neurotheology: Brain, science, spirituality, religious experiences* (pp. 267 –284). San Jose, CA: University Press.

Piacentini, J., & Chang, S. (2001). Behavioral treatments for Tourette syndrome and tic disorders: State of the art. In Cohen, D. J., Jankovic, J., & Goetz, C. G. (Eds.) *Advances in neurology: Tourette syndrome, 85* (pp. 319–332). Philadelphia: Lippincott Williams & Wilkins.

Pikaenen, A., Savander, V., & Le Doux, J. E. (1997). Organization of intra-amygdaloid circuitries in the rat: An emerging framework for understanding functions of the amygdala. *Trends in Neurosciences, 20,* 515–523.

Plato (1974). *The Republic* (E. M. A. Grube, Trans.). Indianapolis, IN: Hackett.

Polster, I., & Polster, M. (1973). *Gestalt therapy integrated.* San Francisco: Jossey-Bass.

Provine, R. (2001). *Laughter: A scientific Investigation.* New York: Penguin Books.

Redmond, D., & Murphy, D. L. (1975). Behavioral correlates of platelet monoamine oxidase (MAO) activity in rhesus monkeys. *Psychosomatic Medicine, 37,* 80.

Reich, W. (1942). *The function of the orgasm.* New York: Orgone Institute.

Reich, W. (1949). *Character analysis.* New York: Noonday.

Reiman, E. M., Fusselman, M. J., Fox, P. T., & Raichle, M. E. (1989). Neuroanatomical correlates of anticipatory anxiety. *Science, 243,* 1071–074.

Richard, P., Moos, F., & Freund-Mercier, M. J. (1991). Central effects of oxytocin. *Physiological Reviews, 71,* 331–370.

Rilling, M. (2000). John Watson's paradoxical struggle to explain Freud. *American Psychologist, 55*(3), 301–312.

Risch, S. C. (1991). *Central nervous system peptide mechanisms in stress and depression.* Washington, DC: American Psychiatry Press.

Robertson, B. L. & Sawyer, C. H. (1957). Loci of sex behavioral and gonadotropic centers in the female cat hippocampus. *Psychologist, 1,* 72.

Rogers, C. M. (1954). Hypothalamic mediation of sex behavior in the male rat. *Unpublished doctoral dissertation,* Yale University, New Haven, CT.

Rogers, R. [Composer], & Hammerstein, O. [Producer] (1951). *The King and I* [Theatrical production] New York, NY; *The King and I* [Film] 1956. United States: Warner Brothers

Roth, B. L. (1994). Multiple serotonin receptors: Clinical and experimental aspects. *Annals of Clinical Psychiatry, 6,* 67–78.

Routtenberg, A. (1978). The reward system of the brain. *Journal of Comparative and Physiological Psychology, 239,* 154–164.

Rozin, P., Lowery, L., Imada, S., & Haidt, J. (1999). The CAD triad hypothesis: A mapping between three moral emotions (contempt, anger, disgust) and three moral codes (community, autonomy, divinity). *Journal of personality and social psychology, 76*(4), 574–586.

Ruffman, T., & Keenan, T. (1996). The belief-based emotion of surprise: The case for a lag in understanding relative to false belief. *Developmental Psychology, 32*(1), 40–49.

Rutledge, T. (2002). *Embracing fear.* Harper: San Francisco.

Sartre, J. P. (1956). *Being and nothingness* (H. Barnes, Trans.). New York: Washington Square Press. (Original work published 1943.)

Sawyer, C. H. (1969). Regulatory mechanisms of secretion of gonadotropic hormones. In W. Haymaker, E. Anderson, & W. J. H. Nauta (Eds.), *The hypothalamus* (pp. 389–430). Springfield, IL: Charles C Thomas.

Schaefer, J., Rutledge. T. (2003). *Life without Ed.* New York: McGraw-Hill.

Schneider, D. (1956). *The image of the heart.* New York: International University Press.

Schwartz, J., & Begley, S. (2002). *The mind and the brain: Neuroplasticity and the power of mental force.* New York: HarperCollins.

Scott, J. P. (1974). Effects of psychotropic drugs on separation distress in dogs. *Exerpta Medic, International Congress Series, 359,* 735–745.

Seneca (1963). *De ira.* Oxford, UK: Loeb Classical Library, Oxford University Press.

Shin, L. M., Dougherty, D. D., Orr, S. P., Pitman, R. K., Lasko, M., Macklin, M. L., Alpert, N. M., Fischman, A. J., & Rauch, S. L. (2000). Activation of anterior paralimbic structures during guilt-related script imagery. *Biological Psychiatry, 48*(1), 43–50.

Siegman, A. W., & Smith, T. W. (1994). *Anger, hostility and the heart.* Hillsdale, NJ: Erlbaum.

Sinha, R., & Parsons, O. A. (1996). Multivariate response patterning of fear and anger. *Cognition and Emotion, 10,* 173–198.

Spinoza, B. (1982). *Ethics.* (S. Shirley, Trans.). Indianapolis, IN: Hackett. (Original work published 1677.)

Sprengelmeyer, R., Young, A., Pundt, I., Sprengelmeyer, A., Calder, A., Berrios, G., Winkel, R., Vollmoeller, W., Kuhn, W., Sartory, G., & Przuntek, H. (1997). Disgust implicated by obsessive-compulsive disorder. *Proceedings of the Royal Society: Biological Sciences, B264,* 1767–1773.

Sprengelmeyer, R., Young, A., Sprengelmeyer, A., Calder, A., Rowland, D., Perrett, D., Homberg, V., & Lange, H. (1997). Recognition of facial expressions: Selective impairment of specific emotions in Huntington's disease. *Cognitive Neuropsychology, 14,* 839–879.

Stampfl, T. G. (1967). Implosive therapy. Part I: The theory. In S. G. Armitage (Ed.), *Behavioral modification techniques in the treatment of emotional disorders.* Battle Creek, MI: V.A. Publications.

Steingard, R., Renshaw, P., Yurgelvn-Todd, D., Appelmans, K., Lyoo, I., Shorrick, K., Bucci, J., Cesena, M., Abebe, D., Zurakowiski, D., Poussaint, T. & Barnes, P. (1996). Structural abnormalities in brain magnetic resonance images of depressed children. *Journal of the American Academy of Child and Adolescent Psychiatry, 35,* 307–311.

Stemmler, G. (1989). The autonomic differentiation of emotions revisited: Convergent and discriminate validation. *Psychophysiology, 26,* 617–632.

Steriade, M., & Amzica, F. (1998). Coalescence of sleep rhythms and their chronology in corticothalamic networks. *Sleep Research Online, 1*(1), 1–10.

Stosny, S. (1995). *Treating attachment abuse: A compassionate approach.* New York: Springer.Strecker, R., Thakkar, M., Porkka-Heiskanen, T., Dauphin, L., Bjorkum, A., & McCarley, R. (1999). Behavioral state-related changes of extracellular serotonin concentration in the pedunculopontine tegmental nucleus: A microdialysis study in freely moving animals. *Sleep Research Online, 2*(2), 21–27.

Strupp, H. (1993). The Vanderbilt psychotherapy studies: Synopsis. *Journal of Consulting & Clinical Psychology, 61*(3), 431–433.

Tangney, J., Miller, R., Flicker, L., & Barlow, D. (1996). Are shame, guilt, and embarrassment distinct emotions? *Journal of Personality and Social Psychology, 70*(6), 1256–1269.

Taub, E., Uswatte, G., & Pidikiti, R. (1999). Constraint-induced movement therapy: a new family of techniques with broad application to physical rehabilitation-a clinical review. *Journal of Rehabilitation Research and Development, 36,* 237–251.

Taylor, S. E. (2001). *The Tending Instinct*. New York: Henry Holt.

Teasdale, J. D., Segal, Z. V., Williams, J. M. G., et al. (2000). Prevention of relapse/recurrence in major depression of mindfulness-based cognitive therapy. *Journal of Consulting & Clinical Psychology, 68*, 615–623.

Teitelbaum, P. (1961). Disturbances of feeding and drinking behavior after hypothalamic lesions. In M. R. Jones (Ed.), *Nebraska Symposium on Motivation* (vol. 9, pp. 39–65). Lincoln: University of Nebraska Press.

Thoits, P. A. (1983). Dimensions of life stress that influence psychological distress. An evaluation and synthesis of the literature. In H. B. Kaplan (Ed.), *Psychological stress: Trends in theory and research* (pp. 33–103). New York: Academic Press.

Tomkins, S. S. (1962). *Affect/imagery/consciousness. Vol. 1: The positive affects.* New York: Springer.

Tomkins, S. S. (1963). *Affect/imagery/consciousness. Vol. 2: The negative affects.* New York: Springer.

Tomkins, S. S. (1981). The quest for primary motives: Biography and autobiography of an idea. *Personality and Social Psychology, 41*, 306–329.

Tucker, D., & Williamson, P. (1984). Asymmetric neural control systems in human self-regulation. *Psychological Review, 91*, 185–215.

Vanderschuren, L., Niesink, R., & Van Ree, J. (1997). The neurobiology of social play behavior in rats. *Neuroscience and Biobehavioral Reviews, 21*, 309–326.

Vaughan, E., & Fisher, A. E. (1962). Male sexual behavior induced by intracranial electric stimulation. *Science, 137*, 758–760.

Watson, J. B. (1970). *Behaviorism* (Rev. ed). New York: Norton. (Original work published 1924.)

Whelton, W., & Greenberg, L. (2000). The self as a singular multiplicity: A process experiential perspective. In C. J. Muran (Ed.), *Self-relations in the psychotherapy process* (pp. 87–106). Washington, DC: American Psychological Association.

Winnicott, D. W. (1989). *Holding and interpretation: Fragment of analysis.* New York: Grove Press.

Wolpe, J., & Rachman, S. (1960). Psychoanalytic evidence: A critique based on Freud's case of Little Hans. *Journal of Nervous and Mental Disease, 131*, 135–145.

Xi, M., Morales, F., & Chase, M. (1999). A GABAargic pontine reticular system is involved in the control of wakefulness sleep. *Sleep Research Online, 2*(2), 43–58.

Yerkes, R. M., & Dodson, J. D. (1908). The relation of strength of stimulus to rapidity of habit-formation. *Journal of Comparative Neurology and Psychology, 18*, 459–482.

About the Author

David W. McMillan, Ph.D. blends his twenty-five years as a clinical psychologist with his in-depth knowledge of emotions to create a fascinating, innovative, and practical book to guide readers on a journey of self-discovery. In both *Emotion Rituals: A Resource for Therapist and Clients* and his previous book, *Create Your Own Love Story*, McMillan simultaneously informs, inspires, and entertains readers as he gives examples of individuals who have incorporated his various therapeutic techniques into their lives.

McMillan's ease in front of an audience makes him an excellent promoter of his books. Not only has McMillan been interviewed on numerous television and radio stations, but he has also hosted his own comedy talk show, "Radio for the Matrimonially Challenged." Additionally, he is comfortable doing presentations and workshops in front of a live audience.

McMillan is internationally recognized as a leader in his field. He is known for the development of the Sense of Community Theory, a cornerstone of Community Psychology Theories. In 1982, he founded the Nashville Psychotherapy Institute. From 1992 to 1997, he chaired the Tennessee Psychological Colleague Association Committee. Currently McMillan is an adjunct faculty member at Vanderbilt University. He is the founder and co-director of both Compose, a program to treat family violence, and of Parkwest Eating Disorder Program.

McMillan is a well-rounded individual whose hobbies include golf, yoga, and Tennessee Titans football. He is married to the Honorable Marietta Shipley, judge of the Davidson County Second Circuit Court. The couple attends Nashville's Second Presbyterian Church. McMillan's primary joy is putting together information into theories that are helpful in the management and understanding of the human experience.

Index

Post-traumatic stress disorder, surprise/
  startle/wonder, 182
Power
  level of, 33–34
  quality of life, 33–34
Praise, 48
Pride, joy, 126
PRIDE ritual
  addiction, 146
    detect pride, 146
    engage life, 146
    identify, 146
    point to, 146
    receive shame, 146
  shame/guilt, 168–170
    detect, 168
    engage life, 168
    inform, 168
    preserve, 168
    receive, 168
Psychological mindedness, 19
Psychological theory
  anatomy, xii
  initial idea, xii
Psychotherapy
  art, integrating, 232–233
  goals, 31
  relationship, 31
  religion, relationship, 3–4
  science, integrating, 232–233

Q

Quality of life, 33
  adolescent, 33–34
  artists, 33
  power, 33–34

R

Reason
  controlling power, 24
  emotion, superiority, 6–7
Reattributing, 38
Refocusing, 38
Rehabilitation, neuroplasticity, 40–42
Relabeling, 38
Relaxation, fear, 28
Relaxation techniques, fear, 93–95
  aerobic exercise, 94
  dead-face trick, 94–95
  friends, family, and pets, 95
  movement, 93–94

physical relaxation tools, 93–94
  stretching, 94
Religion, psychotherapy, relationship, 3–4
Repression, 2
Reptilian brain, 24
Respect, 82
Rest. *see also* Fatigue/rest/trance/sleep
Revaluing, 39
RIGHT ritual
  eating disorder, 47
  obsessive-compulsive disorder, 45–46
Rituals, 4. *see also* Emotion rituals
  benefits, 31–32
  designing, 45–48
  implications for treatment, 237–239
  practice, 34–35
  research on, 36–37
  role, 31–32
  set-up, 35
Rogerian psychotherapy, 3

S

Sadness, 99–112
  ALIVE ritual, 107–110
    awareness, 108
    engage in action, 110
    include faith in process, 109
    learning, 109
    vent, 109–110
  clinical case study, 99–100, 111–112
  compassion, 110–111
  defined, 99
  depression, 102
  emotions resolving, 105–107
  function, 101
  grief, 103–105
  hypothalamus, 61–62
  intelligence, 103
  joy, 129
  limbic system, 100
  medial forebrain, 116
  negative consequences, 101–102
  neurology, 100–101
  neurotransmitters, 101
  periventricular system, 116
  physiology, 101–102
  positive consequences, 102
  surviving loss, 105
Science
  art, integrating, 232–233
  psychotherapy, integrating, 232–233

For Product Safety Concerns and Information please contact our EU representative GPSR@taylorandfrancis.com Taylor & Francis Verlag GmbH, Kaufingerstraße 24, 80331 München, Germany

T - #0094 - 160425 - C0 - 229/152/16 - PB - 9780415861205 - Gloss Lamination